MW00776507

# Qigong

## *A Legacy In Chinese Healing*

# Qigong
## *A Legacy In Chinese Healing*

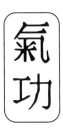

## The Eight Treasures
## With Qigong Meditations

As Presented By

### Dean Y. Deng, M.D.
and
### Enid Ballin, Director

Qigong International ®
New Orleans, LA, USA
Changchun, China

Important Medical Note:
Consult your doctor for medical advice and care.
The information, exercises and procedures presented
in this book are not intended to supersede the
directives of your physician.

Copyright © Dean Y. Deng, M.D. and Enid Ballin, 1998

Library of Congress Catalog Card No. 97-67808

ISBN 0-9657560-8-4
First Edition, First Printing

Printed in the United States of America

Published by Qigong International® Publications

Subsidiary of
Qigong International ®
P.O. Box 56665, New Orleans, LA 70156
In affiliation with Acucenter,  Illinois, U.S.A.

THE EIGHT TREASURES
8
Qigong
International®

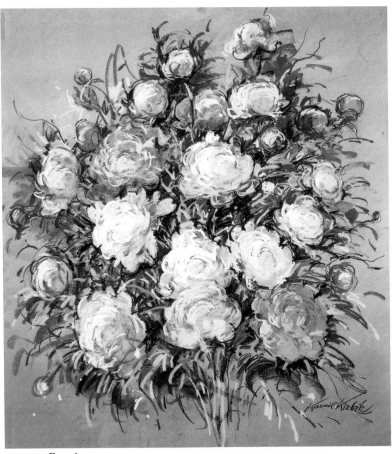

*Peonies*
Kamil Kubik

*Maintaining order rather than correcting
disorder is the ultimate principle of wisdom.*
Emperor Huang Di

Deepest gratitude and respect for my masters, teachers, family and friends shall be forever present within me. To my students and patients who have allowed me the great pleasure and privilege of working with them, thank you. I treasure all of our encounters for they shall continue to enrich my life always.

**Dean Y. Deng, M.D.**

Thank you to my family, my children, Hart and Blair, and to all those who supported me along my path; and to Dr. Deng, whose warmth, generosity, teaching and energy have provided me with a rare and meaningful opportunity with which to repay the love and kindnesses in life.

**Enid Ballin**

ACKNOWLEDGEMENTS

Reproductions from *In the Way of the Master* are used by
permission of The Museum of Fine Arts, Houston, Texas.

"Peonies" Painting by Kamil Kubik

"Lotus" Painting by Li Zhong Hai

Workshop Photographs by Tiejun Shi

Special Photographic work by Bill Cook

Original Editing by
Cary E. Howard, Ph.D.

Final Editing, Composing and Typography
Polly Hanson

Printed by Hauser Printing Co., Inc,
Harahan, LA

# CONTENTS

CONTENTS continued

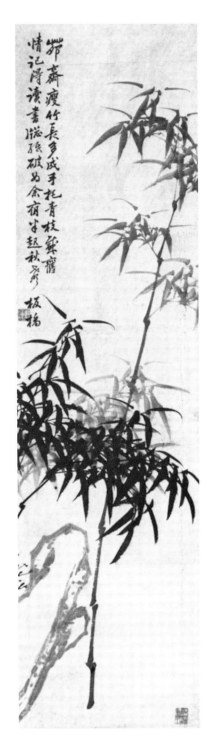

*Bamboo and Rock*
Cheng Hsieh (1693-1765)

# PREFACE

*To be at one with the great law of heaven and earth*
*is to live with purpose, love and dignity.*

From the mists of antiquity comes an extraordinary heritage … the Chinese healing art of Qigong. Qigong (pronounced *chee gong*) was initially developed over five thousand years ago and has enriched the lives of generations over the millennia. Today millions of people in China and around the world continue to practice gentle, relaxing and invigorating Qigong exercises to increase the flow of life energy, or Qi (*chee*), into and throughout their minds and bodies. Their goal, the very principle of Qigong, is to improve health and longevity by cultivating, embracing and directing this vital force toward total life enhancement.

Basically, the simple practice of Qigong involves mental focusing, regulated breathing, established postures and slow body movements. Its versatility creatively molds its almost endless benefits to every individual, regardless of age or health status. Variations may include meditation, self-massage of acupuncture points and meridians and the directing of healing energy or Qi to others.

---

*Qigong, A Legacy in Chinese Healing*, is a special contribution to this field by the highly respected Qigong Master, Dean Y. Deng. One of six children, Dr. Deng was born in China in the Province of Hubei. He is a descendent in a long lineage of Qigong masters, his paternal grandfather being especially well known. At the age of three, Dr. Deng was chosen by an eminent Qigong master in China to receive training in this ancient art. According to Chinese custom, this was a great honor and he had no choice but to practice these powerful techniques everyday. Thus he began to develop his gifts just as many others had done in his distinguished family before him. By the time Dr. Deng was eight years old, he was also receiving regular training in the arts of acupuncture and Kung Fu.

He practiced diligently each day, one exercise being to direct the Qi through his hand to break a stone, a feat Westerners often watch in amazement when demonstrated by martial arts masters. It was "no big deal," he explains, just something that was part of his training. A happy child, he was devoted to helping others. It wasn't until later, while attending medical school, that he learned to fully appreciate the value of emotional control and the importance of mind/body relationship in effectively directing the Qi energy.

One day he became angry with a classmate. At home that evening, the anger of the day lingered as he began to practice breaking the stone. "I didn't break the stone," he laughs, "but I almost broke my hand. It hurt for three weeks!"

Dr. Deng explains that it is the mindful directing of the life energy that provides the force to break a stone or perform other seemingly impossible feats. Negative emotions, especially anger, disrupt the flow of Qi and the force loses its power and effectiveness. This is the reason there is such great emphasis on calming the mind and cultivating positive emotions in Qigong training.

"Although we might not be interested in breaking rocks," Dr. Deng points out, "our own negative thoughts and emotions block the life energy in our bodies and set up the conditions for disease."

Dr. Deng received his medical degree from Sun Yat-Sen University of Medical Sciences, the prestigious and oldest medical school in China. He also served on the University's teaching faculty. In 1988, he received a fellowship to the United States where he began teaching at one of the nation's leading schools of medicine. In subsequent years, he has taught and lectured at several universities in America, China and other countries. He has also conducted innumerable workshops and taught acupuncture in major cities around the world. Dr. Deng is also co-founder of Qigong International® and the Asian American Acupuncture Association.

Dr. Deng maintains a regular healing practice at his

home office in Chicago, Illinois. Widely recognized as an eminent Qigong master, he combines his powerful life experiences with the healing art of acupuncture and traditional Western methodology. By masterfully balancing these skills, Dr. Deng brings a vital integration of East and West to his medical practice.

In addition, Dr. Deng regularly schedules time to teach *The Eight Treasures of Qigong Program*, with associate Enid Ballin. This uniquely designed program was created by Dr. Deng and is based upon his classic Qigong training. He uses and demonstrates his advanced development of Qi to assist students in developing their own energy to maintain mental, physical and spiritual health. Offered internationally, these Qigong healing seminars allow people the world over to share and benefit from Dr. Deng's exceptional insights, training and expertise.

———————————

Enid Ballin, student of meditation and various healing arts for over twenty years, began studying with Dr. Deng in 1991 and became Dr. Deng's Certified Instructor (C.I.E.T) for T*he Eight Treasures of Qigong Program*. Ms. Ballin is also co-founder and Director for Qigong International®.

Her dedication, great enthusiasm and commitment to Qigong, Dr. Deng's work and *The Eight Treasures Program* is based on a foundation of actual experience. She has watched her students' health and energy dramatically improve, as well as her own. Ms. Ballin has witnessed improvements and cures of many illnesses through Dr. Deng's healing work. She has observed scores of individuals in Qigong seminars relieve their pain, reverse illness and restore well-being, many times avoiding hospitalization.

Ms. Ballin explains: "The number of people who travel across the country to see Dr. Deng and attend his seminars attest to his extraordinary success rate in treating all types of diseases and imbalances in the system. He teaches people how to maintain their health through daily practice of these highly beneficial, preventative exercises."

Ms. Ballin, born and educated in New York, has traveled extensively and is fluent in several languages. After moving to New Orleans, Louisiana, she began teaching and coordinating *The Eight Treasures Program* in the area. She then introduced Dr. Deng to New Orleans, where they hold frequent seminars and provide Qigong and acupuncture treatments on a regular basis. Together, they offer this unique program throughout the United States, including Alaska, as well as China and various other locations around the world.

Ms. Ballin also conducts Qigong workshops, private classes and consultations on her own and has presented Qigong in several schools and hospitals. She has made her unique expertise available through special presentation of *The Eight Treasures Program* to passengers of a major cruise line. Traveling with Dr. Deng to China in 1995, Ms. Ballin was invited to lecture at Beijing University of Traditional Chinese Medicine regarding the status of Qigong in America. She returned to China in 1997 where she again gave lectures, classes and demonstrations. She was invited as a guest speaker and presenter at the Second Qigong Conference of Changchun and also conducted a workshop at a major university there. The presentation was taped for Chinese television. Ms. Ballin currently divides her time between homes in Louisiana and China.

Experience confirms that Qigong increases energy, greatly reduces stress and improves the quality of life for those who practice it. It has proven to be instrumental in helping people who are challenged with all types of illness when often Western medicine may fall short. This includes such diseases as cancer, diabetes, arthritis, asthma, immune deficiency and heart disease.

Today government-sponsored Qigong institutes throughout China are engaged in research, teaching and training. Serious research is underway in major universities around the world to further understand the value of Qigong training and acupuncture.

*The Eight Treasures Program* and Meditations presented in this book provide jewels of insight on the development of energy, self-empowerment and health for all who wish to participate. They are designed to promote well-being and happiness. As you practice and enjoy these exercises and techniques, you will experience the special benefits of studying with a foremost Qigong master.

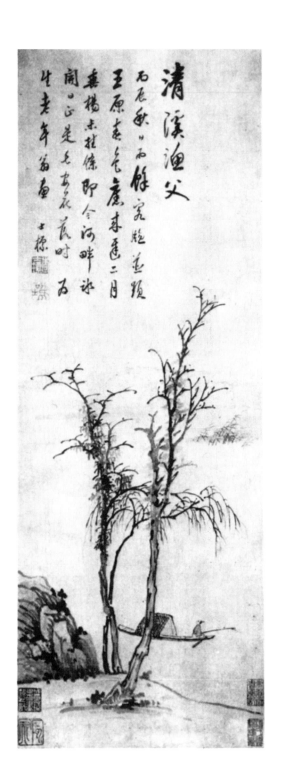

*Old Angler On A Clear Stream*
Ch'a Shih-piao (1615-1698)

*CHAPTER 1*

# THE IMPORTANCE OF QIGONG

Dean Y. Deng, M.D.

*Experience the essence of the life force. Practice and discover The Eight Treasures for yourself.*

## The Life Energy

Qi is the gift of life energy.

Qigong is a gift of fulfillment through Qi.

The ancient Chinese healing art of Qigong (*pronounced chee gong*) is a series of gentle, natural exercises that regulates the flow of Qi, life energy, in the mind and body. Everyone can do it.

Learning and practicing even the basics of the program can result in amazing benefits to health, longevity and total well-being ... and it takes only minutes a day. Defining its essence, Qigong means *practice to develop and*

3

*balance your Qi and be healthy.* It allows one to take direct responsibility for his or her own health and life experience. Everyone has this ability.

The specific origins of Qigong are lost in antiquity, but it is known to date back at least five thousand years. It is not only an important component of traditional Chinese medicine but is, in fact, the basis of all Chinese healing and martial arts and has endured longer than almost all other healing systems.

Qigong has been called a moving meditation. By inviting energy and balance, it creates tranquility through the use of the mind, breath control, easy movements and comfortable postures. Unlike regimens of many other programs of physical fitness and skill development, every Qigong exercise is flexible and supportive of capability. Each movement may be structured, contoured and adapted to meet individual need. Personal comfort is always emphasized because the goal is to increase and enhance the flow of Qi. Never challenge it. Energy manifests simply by access.

The rapidly growing popularity of this extraordinary exercise system is easy to understand. It is simple to do, feels wonderful, increases energy, restores peace of mind and promotes health and general well being. It provides a natural antidote to physical and mental stress. Qigong very often enables the body to cure itself of chronic or debilitating disease and, at the very least, can relieve physical pain and suffering. Unlike drugs, it has no adverse side effects.

In China today, people have a choice between Western

medicine, in which drugs and surgery play an active role, and traditional Chinese medicine, which includes Qigong, acupuncture, herbal medicines and massage. Equal access to both Eastern and Western methodologies are available in hospitals and clinics, allowing the individual to make the choice of treatments they deem most effective. Thus self-responsibility, self-care and a preventive medical approach are primary ingredients in China's contemporary national health care system.

## It Works

Qigong has developed and endured as part of traditional Chinese medicine for one simple reason: it works. As one Qigong master observed, if it didn't work, someone would have noticed by now. There are many diseases and disorders which Western medicine cannot treat effectively but which respond well to and are greatly helped through the practice of Qigong.

When I was an intern finishing my medical training in China, I was completing an academic requirement which called for a medical work-up on one of my professors. As young doctors we were advanced in our knowledge and training, so this seemed like a routine task for me.

I had not yet looked at the chest X-rays and other reports on my professor when I met him in the hall. Teasing him I said, "Well, professor, I'm very sorry to report that you have lung cancer!" Of course, I was only kidding.

But my professor quickly looked at the chart and said, "Dr. Deng, you are right. You have made a fine diagnosis. I do have lung cancer. I didn't know."

Imagine my shock when I actually looked at his X-rays and saw the evidence of cancer in his lungs. He immediately scheduled surgery. Unfortunately, the doctors discovered that it had spread to his spine so they had no recourse but to just sew him back up. The medical diagnosis was that his cancer was beyond treatment and he had only a limited number of months to live. He resigned his post to spend the last few months of his life with his family.

Four years later, when I was seeking letters of reference before leaving for the United States, I returned to the medical school. There in the office stood the professor.

"What are you doing here? You had lung cancer!" I blurted out, amazed that he was still alive but overjoyed to see him. I told him who I was, and he said, "Oh yes, Dr. Deng, you are a fine doctor. You diagnosed my lung cancer."

I said that I might be a fine doctor, but I obviously didn't know what to do for his lung cancer. So what had he done?

He told me that he had tried a little chemotherapy and radiation, but I knew those treatments didn't help much with his kind of cancer. So I asked what else he had done, because all of us knew he was beyond medical help.

He explained that after he had returned home, he went to see a Qigong master. He received healing treatments and began practicing Qigong everyday. He soon began to feel better and stronger. When I saw this man again four years later, he was still healthy! Since that time, the cancer has remained under control and he continues living an active, productive life.

## Qigong and Energy Medicine

Although I had been practicing Qigong since I was a young child, I only began to realize the power behind this ancient healing art as I matured. Several months before coming to live in the United States, various people who were aware of my Qigong training asked for help with physical problems. These ranged from sore muscles and headaches to serious stomach problems. I directed Qi to each of them to help get the energy flowing through their bodies. Not only did they get great relief but the disorders completely cleared up. I realized that practicing Qigong and projecting and directing the flow of life energy was an integrative tool in both Eastern and Western medical approaches. This, in fact, is the essence of the emerging field of energy medicine. The Qi or life energy sustains and heals us. Balancing the life force within the body enables us to receive the energy we need to heal ourselves.

You probably have heard the old saying, *The doctor may treat the wound, but the body heals itself.* This recognizes the importance of the regenerative energy that is needed for healing and life itself.

When a person's condition is too weak or depleted

7

to mobilize the body's forces to correct an imbalance or disease, one must then turn to outside forces. In traditional Chinese medicine this has been accomplished through the use of medicinal herbs, massage, acupuncture, and/or direct emission of energy from healer to patient.

Everyone has ability to develop, balance and direct the life force. Qigong is the simplest and most effective practice which enables us do this for ourselves. We are all healers of self and others if we but awaken our knowledge and awareness of this potential.

Every individual case is different, of course, and no blanket claims can be made. The state of advancement of a disorder and one's receptivity to Qi play a part. We realize that, just like the yin and the yang, life and death are part of our total experience. None of us can escape death, but hopefully we can walk through life with minimum physical problems and discomfort and max-imum awareness and vitality. Regardless of our stage of life or our level of wellness, practicing the gentle techniques of Qigong can help restore a feeling of inner peace and well-being.

The government supported Qigong Institute in Beijing (Fig.1.0) is engaged in extensive Qigong research. Patients receive healing treatments from Qigong prac-titioners as well as instruction in Qigong practice. Professionals engaged in the healing arts are also trained in Qigong as preventive health care. Other healing therapies include acupuncture, massage, and herbal remedies.

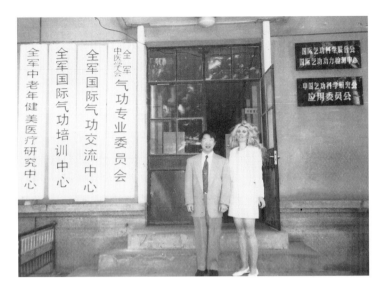

*Figure 1.0  Dr. Dean Y. Deng and Enid Ballin visiting the Qigong Institute in Beijing, China – 1995*

In this and many similar institutes in China, people learn self-care methods to address such conditions as muscle, back and joint pain, daily stress, poor circulation, constipation, fatigue, immune disorders, cancer and hypertension. Ongoing research is aimed at gaining a greater scientific knowledge of Qi and ascertaining how best to treat a wide range of disorders.

Today, Qigong is being tested in research laboratories around the world and is now a subject being studied by Western medicine. Interest in learning and practicing Qigong has increased greatly throughout the United States and other countries, especially since a greater number of Qigong masters have begun traveling, sharing their knowledge and greatly expanding their teaching base.

## The Eight Treasures Program

In this book, I am happy to offer you a simple, yet powerful program you can perform in only 15 minutes a day. It has evolved from my years of study and training in classic Qigong. It includes five preparation exercises and nine focused arm movements. The movements and breathing exercises are gentle, patterned after nature and can be done by anyone at any age, regardless of health status. You may perform these exercises in a sitting or standing position, or even reclining if you are weak and recovering from illness. You may wear whatever attire you wish.

This program develops your Qi, your life force, and reveals and enhances your body's own capacity for healing itself. In addition, I have offered four special meditation exercises which will strengthen and develop the major energy channels of your body, your internal organs, and improve your health and vitality.

The medical benefits of Qigong can be realized in a surprisingly short period of time. Through relaxed, calm movement, breathing and concentration, blocked energy is released, allowing it to flow smoothly through the body's meridians. I have been very pleased to see many wonderful results in my patients and students.

There is the story told of a great master who had reached a very old age. It was now his time to die and his sad students gathered around him. They asked for one last insightful teaching that would bring them comfort and guidance. What was his great secret to health, happiness, longevity and mastership? He smiled as he departed this world and whispered only one word: "P-r-a-c-t-i-c-e."

Practice Qigong and it will work for you. That's the reason we wrote this book. We dedicate these pages to your full enjoyment of life and all of its experiences, encounters and lessons and to your spiritual, mental and physical health.

Remember, all it takes is practice.

Qi (Life Energy)

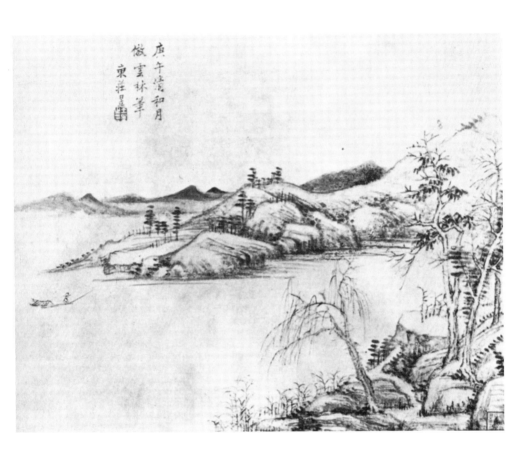

*Landscape in the Style of Ni Tsan, 1690*
Wang Yu (1662-1722)

*CHAPTER 2*

# THE HISTORY
# AND MEANING
# OF QIGONG

*Before creation a presence existed, self-contained,*
*complete, formless, changeless ... I call it the Tao.*
– Lao-Tzu –

## Ancient Roots In Taoist Philosophy

The history of Qigong reaches back 5000 years. Its roots originate in early Taoism (*pronounced Dow-ism*) although no one is certain when the concept of life energy, or Qi, actually emerged. Taoism was well known for centuries and further developed through the wisdom of an ancient sage, Lao-Tzu. Lao-Tzu is believed to have been born around 604 B.C.E. His name translates as "Old Master" or "Old Boy," titles of great respect and esteem which surround this legendary figure.

It is said that Lao-Tzu became disenchanted when people failed to grasp the simplicity of living in harmony with the Tao, developing the natural energy and goodness within themselves. When asked to record his profound knowledge for the sake of helping others, Lao-Tzu wrote some of his teachings before riding off on a water buffalo in search of seclusion. These teachings, called the *Tao Te Ching*, or *Way of Life*, are the heart of the Taoist philosophy. They were left for the people to interpret on their own because Lao-Tzu never returned.

In Chinese philosophy the Tao is the law of heaven and earth. The Tao is the great unitive principle of all life and basically means that everything is energy.

Loosely translated Tao means *the Way*. It is the way of ultimate reality, the great unseen life force from which all things emerge and to which all things return. The Tao Te Ching says, *"Conceived as having no name, it is the origin of heaven and earth. Conceived as having a name, it is the mother of all things."* The Tao is the great cosmic principle of life, comprising seen and unseen, form and formless, finite and infinite. It includes all time and space – past, present and future, manifesting and transcending the illusion of life and death.

The Tao has been called many names in many cultures: Absolute, Energy, Brahman, Great Spirit, Supreme Design, Universal Order, Universal Being, Divine Mind, God, Unknowable and Nameless One.

Taoism emphasizes simplicity in living and being in harmony with nature. Just as the seasons come and go in a continuing process of birth, growth, decay and death, (spring, summer, fall and winter, respectively) so too are all forms and events cyclic. All emerges and returns to Tao, mother and father of creation, after a brief display on life's stage.

The ancient Taoists did not have much use for aggressive behavior, competition, and extravagance. They emphasized emotional calm and respect for others.

They practiced quelling negative emotions and maintained physical cleanliness for health. A pure, calm, clear mind was necessary to attune to the cosmic source, wellspring of health and longevity. (Fig 2.0, the ancient Taoist Nostrum for curing all ailments.)

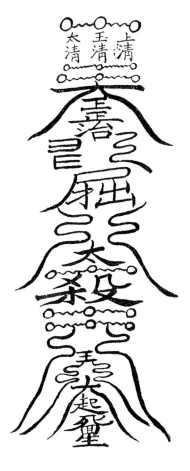

Figure 2.0 Ancient Taoist
Nostrum For Curing
All Ailments.

The Taoists do not see themselves as separate from life's great Reality, but woven into its very fabric. There are no gods to appease, no absolutes, no original sin or falling away from goodness. Through *awareness* of Tao, the core of all being, one learns to receive and exchange energy and wisdom for guidance in everyday life. If you open body, mind and spirit to the presence of Tao, the life energy or Qi, you feel tranquility and peace within yourself and with the world.

The basic Taoist teachings are concerned with how to live in harmony with the life force, achieving health, wisdom and longevity. One cannot fully comprehend the Tao, of course, because it is beyond the capacity of what modern society accepts as a rational mind. Yet through *training and developing awareness* one can intuitively experience the Way, flowing with its power in daily life.

## The Yin and the Yang

Taoism and Chinese philosophy recognize two polar forces, yin and yang, which emerge from and return to the depths of Tao. The life force is the source and support of yin and yang; the three are one great process of energy. The symbol of the Trinity, two emerging from the One, is found in many philosophic and religious traditions.

Everything consists of yin and yang. The dual powers are responsible for the diversity of creation: appearance of all phenomena, processes and changes in the universal drama. (Fig. 2.1, Yin/Yang Symbol.)

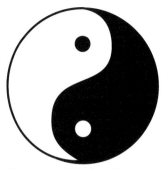

*Figure 2.1 Yin/Yang Symbol*

The yin and yang represent how things come into being and pass away, how the world of seeming opposites exists. It is said that Heaven was created by an abundance of yang and Earth by an abundance of yin. The yin/yang polarity is represented by such polar opposites as female-male, earth-heaven, stillness-movement, yielding-firm, cold-hot, dark-bright, night-day, low-high, down-up, left-right, passive-active, negative charge-positive charge and so on.

In the human body, it is essential that the yin and yang forces be balanced in every organ, system and process to maintain health. From the cellular level of the body to the far reaches of the universe, yin and yang exist in dynamic interaction. When balance is maintained, all things follow a definite order and flow smoothly.

Yet, within every yang force is some yin and within every yin force is some yang. The Chinese symbol of the two pear shaped bodies in a circle represents the two forces emerging from the one life principle, each containing the seed of the other. Eight trigrams of broken and unbroken lines, their origins unknown, were also developed to represent the pairs of opposites and continual changes in the universal order.

These were combined with the yin and yang symbol to form the *Pa Kua* (Fig. 2.2). This exists as the essential foundation of the Chinese *I Ching*, or *Book of Changes*, one of the oldest and most significant books in world literature. The *Pa Kua* in primal arrangement represents the complementary forces responsible for all creation.

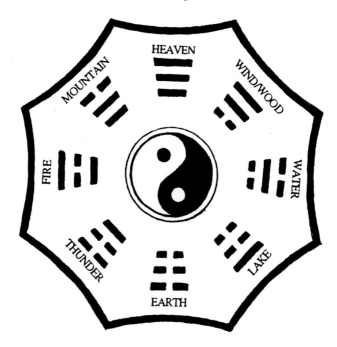

*Figure 2.2. The Pa Kua in primal arrangement. The 8 trigrams, as pairs of complementary opposites, surround the pear shaped yin and yang symbols contained in a circle. In the I Ching, the trigrams and their combinations reflect all possible conditions and processes for change in the universe. It is said we should contemplate the meaning of yin and yang, emerging from and returning to the Tao in cyclic oneness. In this way, we may begin to realize that all life is part of one great energy.*

The way of the yin and yang is also called the way of the left and the right. A simple example is that the left side of your body cannot exist without the right side, and both are a part of one another. The key word in understanding interplay of yin and yang is *balance*. This concept of balancing the yin and yang, being in harmony with the Tao, gave birth to Qigong.

## The Meaning of Qigong

The forces of body, mind and spirit flow from the Tao and are part of it. Qi is the unlimited reservoir of energy that flows everywhere throughout the universe and sustains all life. It is the life spirit energizing your mind and body and the life tool of the universe. It is formless and enlivens and sustains all forms. You might think of Qi as an electrical current lighting up the intelligence and proper functioning of every cell, tissue, organ, system and energy meridian in the body.

The Chinese characters representing *Qi* and *gong* are difficult to translate into English but they do shed light on the meaning of this ancient art (Fig. 2.3).

Basically, Qi means the *life force energy*. The Chinese character for *Qi* translates as *human being lies down on the earth, under the sky and universe and breathes the air and eats the rice*. This is how we receive and sustain the vital life force in our bodies: we get rest, breathe fresh air and eat good food. Qi is also seen as the bioelectric energy or internal energy that maintains our physical and mental well-being.

21

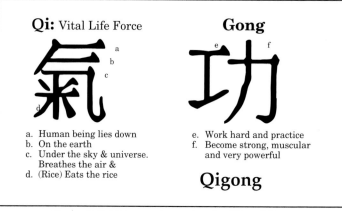

*Figure 2.3 Chinese characters for Qi and Gong.*

The Chinese character for *gong* loosely translates as *work hard and practice and become strong and powerful*. In the Chinese language, *gong* (sometimes shown as *kung*) can also mean achievement, merit and good results. It symbolizes the manifestation of power through the movements of the body, or manifesting your external power.

The combined characters of *Qigong* suggest practicing the art of developing internal and external power and balancing the internal energy with the external energy. This is the secret to maintaining vitality. One must develop and nurture the internal energy, use it, then return it to the universe.

The ancient Chinese quite naturally were concerned with developing energy and strength. They lived in an often harsh environment and were subjected to difficult life conditions. Finding sources for strength and vitality were necessary in order to survive. Thus, from its earliest beginnings Qigong was a healing art. The people of antiquity discovered that certain movements, perhaps through dancing or stretching, certain ways of breathing, and certain ways of massaging and holding the body produced reliable therapeutic results. Not only did they improve vitality and physical strength, but they relieved ailments and disease.

Over several millennia these emerged into definite sets of movements and breathing exercises, with thousands of variations. Understanding the Qi and the balance of yin and yang within the body was the foundation of all Chinese healing practices, including herbal therapy, massage, and acupuncture. Described as *acupuncture without needles*, Qigong is considered one of the highest forms of healing in China today, just as it was thousands of years ago.

In China, teaching and learning Qigong was reserved for men and passed down from generation to generation. It has only been in modern times that Qigong has been widely available to Chinese women. The men of old were protective of these vital secrets for health and strength, not recognizing the importance of sharing their knowledge.

Different types of Qigong have developed based upon varying need and philosophy. Medical Qigong, part of today's traditional Chinese medicine, focuses on healing self *and others*. Confucian Qigong focuses on an *individual's* practice to regulate mind, maintain health and cultivate virtue; Taoist Qigong focuses on physical longevity and secrets of immortality; Buddhist Qigong is designed to purify and ultimately guide the practitioner to universal oneness.

## The Martial Arts

A widely accepted view in China is that Qigong is the oldest of the martial arts and is the foundation upon which all other forms evolved. It might actually be called the art of self-protection against disease, imbalance and disorder. It was said that if one could master Qigong, one could master any area of life and become a master in any other martial art. Qigong was used to increase strength and direct power to the muscles in other martial arts .

A similar discipline emerging from Qigong is Tai Chi. Both are known as "soft" arts because they develop internal energy and are concerned with health and well-being. They overlap in theory and methods. Tai Chi, which grew out of Qigong, is practiced for general balance and harmony. The movements are more structured, intricate and dance-like and require detailed learning. Qigong places emphasis on calming the mind, receiving, experiencing and strengthening internal Qi and developing the ability to emit Qi energy. It focuses on helping the student design his or her own pattern for energy development, receiving the life force through the "thought of no thought."

Kung Fu, a popular martial art in the West, develops external or "hard" energy for fighting. However, development of internal or "soft" Qi is needed to have an increased supply of life force to strengthen the muscles and aid speed of movement.

China's history is filled with amazing feats by Qigong masters and, even today, they are widely known for their strength and imperviousness to injury and pain. Through mental focusing, a master can make himself virtually invulnerable and if he is ill or wounded can quickly heal himself. A master's energy is just as powerful in healing others if he chooses to use it in this way.

Every movement and posture assumed in Qigong or any martial art form has the balanced elements of the yin and yang. One learns to flow with the Tao, to use all forces, not resist them. It is said that a tranquil mind can anticipate in advance all movements of another. Once one has learned fully to apply the principles of yin and yang, he has mastered his art.

## Qigong and Yoga

Almost every culture has devised and developed ways by which to align with the life force. Some achieve this through meditation, others through movement, breathing, visualization, ritual, dance, prayer and/or song. One system which shares many similarities to Qigong is Yoga. Yoga emerged from the Hinduism and Buddhism tradition in ancient India while Qigong was founded on Chinese medicine, Taosim, Confucianism, Buddhism and the martial arts. Both systems date back thousands of years and promote peace of mind, well-being and longevity.

The Western world has been more familiar with Yoga than Qigong mostly due to accessibility. Historically, China has always been more isolated, with centuries of internal strife and upheaval. Its population has been remote, having to concentrate almost solely on survival. Yoga, on the other hand, found its way westward over three decades ago and was soon embraced by a society more than willing to accept a newly introduced concept. It has been only relatively recent, within the decade of the 90's, that Qigong began to emerge and gain the attention of the West.

Qigong and Yoga share many common points in principal and training technique but differ in philosophical background and procedure.

Similarities derive from the fact that both work with the body's energy systems. Each emphasizes relaxation, concentration, meditation, breathing, postures and movements.

Both Qigong and Yoga are effective systems working toward a common goal of well-being but their paths to achievement are quite different. Qigong is based on sensing and directing Qi and accessing the body meridians, the location of Qi cavities in the body. Emphasis is on the balancing of yin and yang. Yoga's understanding and focus is on the body's chakras (energy centers).

The practice of Qigong, as typified by The Eight Treasures Program, presents no physical extremes, requiring only a relaxed mind, regulated breathing and gentle movements. Yoga postures can be more complex, physically demanding and may involve more strenuous stretching of the body, particularly concentrating on agility and flexibility of the spine.

In Qigong, a healthy diet is recommended but is not limited to vegetarian foods. Often the Yoga practitioner is encouraged to follow only a vegetarian diet.

Qigong is based upon receptivity to the Qi, sensing and allowing it to flow through the body. The practitioner does the exercises, *allowing the energy to flow throughout his or her being*, then *moves* it where it is needed. In other words, one invites the Qi and directs the natural flow of energy. With more advanced training, Qigong may also include self massage for self healing, as well as learning to emit Qi as healing energy to others. Most forms of Yoga do not emphasize massage and lean more toward internalizing benefits rather than sending healing energy.

Like Qigong, many variations of Yoga exist and have been developed over thousands of years for specific applications. For example, in China today, there are numerous types of Qigong, each a definitive sub-division of the whole, created to address a particular objective. *The Eight Treasures of Qigong Program*, presented in these pages, includes exercises and postures which serve as a foundation for all and provide the practitioner with a basic knowledge of how to achieve the greatest benefits from an extraordinary self-fitness and healing art.

As in religious Qigong, the goal of Hindu and Buddhist Yoga is enlightenment or Buddhahood. However, based on the premise of first things first, Taoist Qigong works with the life energy in the body to promote longevity.

The Taoists recognized that one needed to be healthy and live long enough to be able to achieve that desired enlightenment and expanded awareness.

## The Mystery and Mastery of Qi

In Qigong, one trains the body and mind to flow with the life force and to balance the yin and yang. This accomplishes much, including making you feel good.

The Western mind is conditioned to think more in terms of God rather than life force. There is no conflict. God takes care of you, but you heal yourself through awareness and use of this inner and outer power always available to you. It is part of your gift of life. You have the wisdom of the universe ready to serve you *and*, so important to understand, *you are an integral part of that wisdom.*

We must always be willing to invite possiblity ... to expand our perspectives and visions in order to maximize our awareness and capabilities. Only then can we truly improve the qualilty of our lives. We must open doors and rediscover old treasures as well as explore the new.

Opening the door to Qigong and learning to direct the Qi means consciously working with the most powerful force in the universe. The potential is timeless and limitless.

As you practice the art of Qigong and become more and more attuned to the flow of Qi, you will rediscover the true source of energy, health, and wholeness. The better we know ourselves, the easier it is to overcome ignorance and fear, our greatest enemies.

We can take responsibility for our lives. When we are in harmony with the Tao, we can let go of control and be at one with the universe for a life of personal freedom, health and happiness.

Eternity

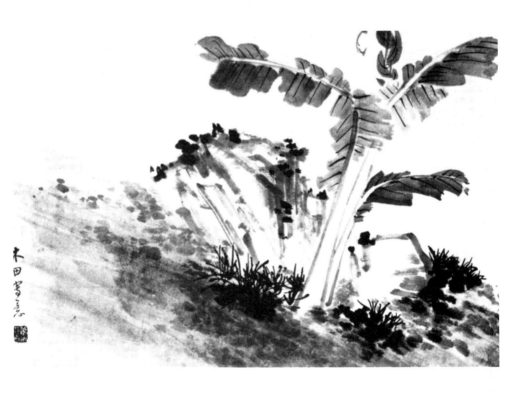

*Banana Palm*
Li Fang-Ying  (1695-1754)

# CHAPTER 3

# YOUR BODY AND ENERGY MERIDIANS

*My way is so simple to feel, so easy to apply,*
*that only a few will feel it or apply it.*

– Lao-Tzu –

## The Electric Body

Your body is a vast network of energy fields and has its own bioelectric frequency. To better vizualize it, think of your body as a local web site, sending and receiving messages constantly with the universal web.

The Chinese have sought for thousands of years to further understand this system of energy. Although they could not see it, they could feel and experience it. Some individuals *are* able to see these finer energy fields, especially when they develop the third eye energy, but most of us have yet to awaken that sensitivity.

Our physical eyes cannot see many energies, waves and rays that exist, because they are beyond our visual spectrum: radio and television waves, microwaves, ultraviolet and infrared waves, X-rays, electromagnetic waves, brain waves, etc. Today's technology allows us to track, measure and graph many of them with highly sensitive instruments. There is now also some specialized instrumentation that can detect and measure the amount of Qi emitted by a person, most especially the masters and others adept in the practice of Qigong.

We do know that the amount of energy and its balance in one's system determines vitality and health. Most of us can look at someone's skin tone, brightness of the eyes and general demeanor or presence and tell whether he or she is feeling up or down or has high or low energy. This is not particularly unusual. It is familiar and something we do quite naturally.

Whether we realize it or not, we constantly monitor energy fields within and around us, especially other people's energy levels. Our whole mind/body system depends upon the continuing exchange, balance and support from the life force and our awareness and interaction with others.

## Energy Meridians

The ancient Chinese discovered great circles or meridians of energy flowing through the body. In traditional Chinese medicine there are twelve primary

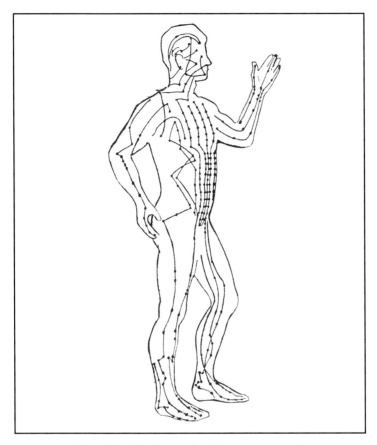

*Figure 3.0 The human body is a vast network
of energy channels or meridians.*

channels for regulating the organs, eight extraordinary vessels, some fifteen accompanying channels, and many other smaller meridians.

Although no one knows for certain, it is estimated there are 71 known energy meridians and over 570 recognized energy cavities or acupuncture points, but more are continuously being discovered. (Fig. 3.0)

This connective energy web supplies power to the

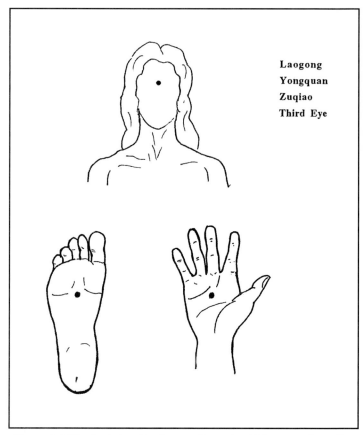

Laogong
Yongquan
Zuqiao
Third Eye

*Figure 3.1 The body has 5 gateways through which energy is easily exchanged with the environment; palms of the hands (laogong cavity), soles of the feet (yongquan cavity) and the third eye.*

system, connects our consciousness to the outside world, and determines our awareness of the universal order. In addition there are five openings or gateways in the body where energy is easily exchanged with the environment and helps balance the Qi. These are the two cavities in the center of the palms (*laogong*), the cavities in the center of the balls of the feet (*yongquan*), and the third eye area (Fig. 3.1).

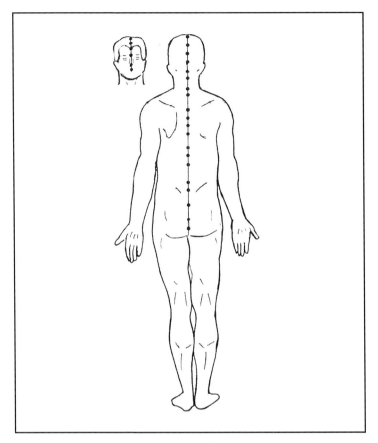

*Figure 3.2 Du Mai, the Governing Vessel*

The two most important vessels or meridians in Qigong training are called the *Governing Vessel* or Du Mai (Fig. 3.2) and the *Conception Vessel* or Ren Mai (Fig. 3.3). These two channels comprise the *microcosmic orbit*. It is said that when the microcosmic orbit is open and balanced, one experiences complete wellness. There is no illness or disharmony within the physical, mental, emotional, and spiritual systems.

The Governing Vessel runs from the base of the spine

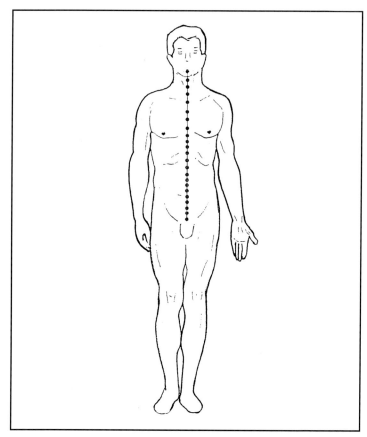

Figure 3.3 Ren Mai, the Conception Vessel

to the top of the head and down to the third eye between the eyebrows. It rejuvenates the spinal fluids and neurological pathways, energizes the brain and increases alertness and mental clarity. The Conception Vessel runs along the front of the body from the perineum to the head. It promotes the healthy functioning of the respiratory and digestive organs by supplying ample energy for balance and efficiency.

The Governing and Conception Vessels connect in the

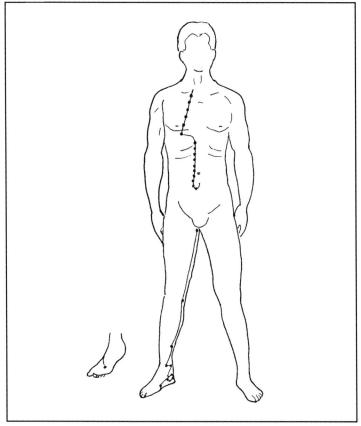

*Figure 3.4 The kidney meridian of the foot and leg*

mouth. This connection is enhanced during Qigong practice by lightly touching the tip of the tongue to the upper palate slightly behind the front teeth.

These two vessels, plus the twelve primary channels, make up the fourteen classic meridians. This is called the *heavenly orbit* or cycle. The Governing and Conception Vessels supply Qi to the lesser meridians and nourish the organs and systems of the body. The Governing Vessel controls the yang channels and the Conception Vessel regulates the yin (including stomach)

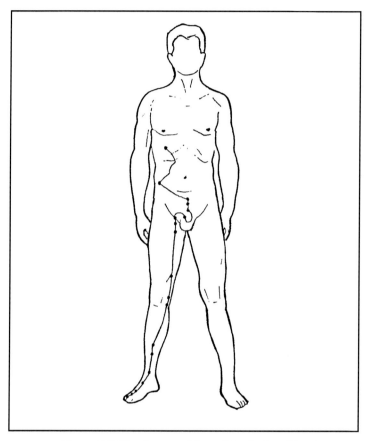

*Figure 3.5 The liver meridian of the foot and leg*

channels.

We actually work with the total system whenever we move energy through the body. Points and channels may vary slightly from person to person, just as we observe the variation of biological characteristics. In The Eight Treasures and Meditation exercises, we work a great deal with the Governing and Conception Vessels because they determine our good health. We also work specifically with the kidney meridian (Fig. 3.4) and

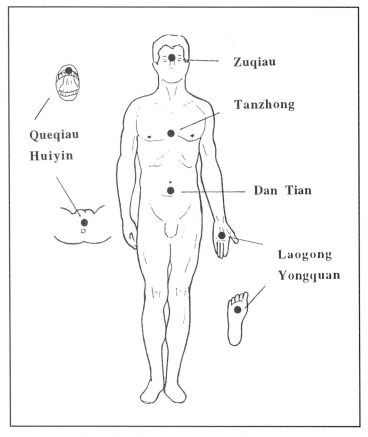

*Figure 3.6 Key energy centers, front view*

liver meridian (Fig. 3.5) which follow upward along the inner leg.

Other than understanding that there are major meridians and key energy centers (Figs. 3.6 and 3.7) along the pathways, it is not necessary to memorize a lot of information. The important thing is moving the Qi through your body. It will travel through its own best pathways and correct any imbalances.

41

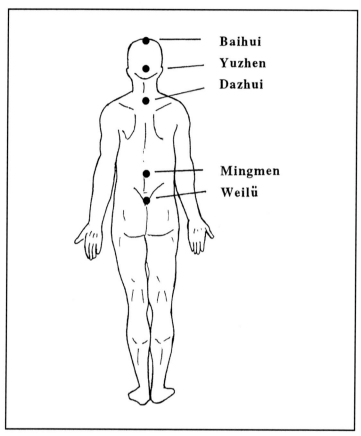

Figure 3.7 Key energy centers, back view

## The Triple Warmer and the Dan Tian

Another major area of focus in the Qigong program is called the triple warmer (or the triple burner – it goes by several names). These are lower, middle and upper areas of the body. The triple warmer is considered to be a yang "organ" although it is actually comprised of several metabolic centers which include various organs.

These same general areas contain three primary Qi cavities or reservoirs called the lower, middle and upper Dan Tian (which means *elixir field*). These are reservoirs or fields of the elixir, or the Qi energy.

The *lower warmer* is located in the lower abdominal region, beginning below the navel, and includes the kidneys and urinary bladder. Two to three inches below the navel and one to two inches inside the body is the first great reservoir of Qi called the lower Dan Tian. Developing awareness of this area and building its reservoir of power is central to all martial arts training. The Japanese term for mentally shaping or guiding the Qi is Ki (pronounced key). Sometimes we use this term Ki when referring to the lower Dan Tian when our intent is to focus the mind and direct Qi throughout various meridians.

The *middle warmer* is located between chest and navel, including the stomach, liver and spleen. It houses the *middle Dan Tian* (Shan Zhong or Tanzhong) which is located between the nipples.

The *upper warmer* includes the chest, neck, head, brain and the functions of the heart and lungs. It houses the *upper Dan Tian (Baihui)* on the top of the head. The *Baihui* is a very powerful center. Its meaning suggests the meeting or convergence of 100 energies. You might think of it as a great cosmic convention center, where all energy meridians meet and Heaven's bounty pours into the human system.

Some exercises for directing Qi through these vital areas include mental focusing, clasping the hands and raising the arms over the head, then slowly bringing them down. This increases Qi, nourishes the organs, stretches, massages and relaxes internal muscles.

# The Body's Organs

Perhaps you have heard someone ask in jest, "How's your liver today?" instead of "How are you doing?" This comes from an old practice of linking the organs with emotional states as well as with biological functions. In Chinese medicine there are five primary paired yin and yang organs.

Although not specific organs, the pericardium (yin) and the triple warmer (yang) are also considered organs, bringing the total to six each. Often a discussion of these areas includes the pericardium as part of the heart and describes the triple warmer under general physiological functions.

## YIN ORGANS

The yin organs are the heart, pericardium, lungs, liver, spleen and kidneys. They produce, store and regulate Qi, blood and fluids in the body. (See The Five Elements chart Fig 3.8.)

*THE HEART: (The heart regulates the emotion of joy and is associated with summer, the color red, a bitter taste, and is paired with the small intestine.)*

Located in the chest cavity, the heart regulates the blood vessels and the flow of blood, in addition to holding the position of ruler in the body. The Chinese believe that the heart is the root of consciousness and spiritual intelligence, and that the mind is really a higher energy field of the heart. The heart regulates all mental functioning. When the heart Qi is balanced, cognitive thinking and memory will be sharp and clear, emotions stabilized, and sleep patterns rejuvenated.

**PERICARDIUM:** The membranous sac enclosing the heart is a very important area in Qigong training. Its function is to regulate the flow of Qi in and around the heart and to dissipate excess Qi caused by emotional turmoil, illness or too much exercise. It helps reduce fever and restore balance. It directs excess Qi to the acupuncture point (laogong cavity) in the center of the palm where it is naturally released. The pericardium is paired with the triple warmer.

**LUNGS:** (*The lungs regulate the emotion of grief. Deep, healthy breathing patterns promote a relaxed, tranquil attitude. The lungs are associated with the autumn season, the color white, a pungent taste, and are paired with the large intestine.*) Located in the chest, the lungs regulate respiration and the flow of Qi throughout the entire body. Through inhalation they bring Qi into the system and push it throughout the body, and then exhale impurities. The lungs also help control flow of fluids through their rhythmic movements, govern the sweat glands and help nourish the skin and the growth of body hair.

**LIVER:** (*The liver regulates the emotion of anger. It is associated with the spring season, the color green, a sour taste*

45

Figure 3.8 The Five Elements

In Chinese philosophy everything is made up of the five elements, which are better understood as forces, powers or aspects emerging from the Tao. These five elements are inherent in all things and symbolize interrelated functions and processes.

Water is linked with that which has declined and is ready for growth; Wood symbolizes that which is growing or expanding; Earth reflects balance and equality; Fire represents a high state preparing to decrease; and Metal suggests declining and decay.

Each of the five elements has its special correspondences with organs of the body, seasons of the year, smells, colors, tastes, and so on. See the chart below.

Also see Five Elements Diagram on page 52.

|  | WATER | WOOD | EARTH | FIRE | METAL |
|---|---|---|---|---|---|
| Yin Organ | Kidneys | Liver | Spleen | Heart | Lung |
| Yang Organ | Urinary Bladder | Gall Bladder | Stomach | Small Intestine | Large Intestine |
| Color | Black | Green | Yellow | Red | White |
| Sound | Groan | Shout | Sing | Laugh | Weep |
| Smell | Rotten | Musty | Fragrant | Burnt | Rancid |
| Taste | Salty | Sour | Sweet | Bitter | Pungent |
| Opening | Ears | Eyes | Mouth | Tongue | Nose |
| Tissue | Bones | Sinews | Flesh | Blood Vessels | Skin/Hair |
| Emotion | Fear | Anger | Sympathy | Joy | Grief |
| Animal | Bear | Deer | Monkey | Bird | Tiger |
| Season | Winter | Spring | Late Summer | Summer | Autumn |
| Climate | Cold | Wind | Dampness | Heat | Dryness |
| Process | Storage | Birth | Transform | Growth | Harvest |

*and is paired with the gall bladder.)*

The liver is located in the upper lateral abdominal region, below the ribs. It governs bile secretions, helps regulate digestion and acts in the formation and movement of blood and Qi flow. It assists in the metabolism of fats, carbohydrates, proteins, vitamins and minerals, helping to nourish the body and promote nail growth. When we do not control anger, the Qi is interrupted and we lose our essential power. Not only do we lose external effectiveness, but internal Qi is blocked and we can quickly set up the conditions for illness.

**SPLEEN:** *(The spleen regulates the emotion of sympathy, and is associated with late summer, the color yellow, a sweet taste, and is paired with the stomach.)*

The spleen lies on the left side, below the diaphragm, in the upper abdominal region. It absorbs nutrients and water and transports them to the lungs and heart. It helps keep the blood circulating and strengthens the muscles. It filters and stores blood and thus is a transformer and transporter of nourishing elements in blood and Qi. It aids in the production of saliva, nourishes the lips and promotes a healthy appetite.

**KIDNEYS:** *(The kidneys regulate the emotion of fear. They are associated with the season of winter, the color black, a salty taste and are paired with the urinary bladder.)*

The kidneys are located on each side of the spine in the lower back region. They regulate growth and development through the storage of Qi. They produce marrow for the bones, brain and spinal column, and help the lungs distribute Qi. They regulate body water and excrete metabolic wastes in the form of urine. They provide Qi to the ear and maintain healthy hearing. The health of the kidneys is considered primary in the overall well being of the individual.

## YANG ORGANS

The yang organs include the small intestine, San Jiao or triple warmer, large intestine, stomach, gall bladder and urinary bladder.

*SMALL INTESTINE: (Like the heart, the small intestine is associated with joy and happiness, the color red, a bitter taste, and is related to summer.)*

The small intestine is located in the abdomen, consists of the duodenum, jejunum and the ileum. It is paired with the heart. It stores, digests and passes on the food it receives from the stomach. It plays an important role in separating wastes from nutrients and passing on wastes to the large intestine. It cleanses and provides Qi energy to the entire system.

*SAN JIAO: San Jiao* means triple warmer and is paired with the pericardium. It includes the areas from the lower abdomen to the brain. Although it is not a specific organ it serves an overall vital function: the upper warmer, through a synthesis of processes including the heart and lungs, sends blood and Qi throughout the whole body. The middle warmer integrates the processes of the spleen and stomach to absorb and utilize the nutrients and the Qi. The lower warmer regulates the storage of Qi, water metabolism, and excretion of liquid wastes.

**LARGE INTESTINE:** *(The large intestine is linked with grief or sadness, the color white, a pungent taste, and the season of autumn.)*

Located in the abdomen, the large intestine forms an arch around the convolutions of the small intestine and extends from the ileum to the anus. It is paired with the lungs. Its primary function is the metabolism of water and excretion of wastes. It extracts water from solid waste material, sends it on to the urinary bladder, then excretes the remaining wastes as stool. It is important that Qi circulate freely in the intestines so that wastes do not become stagnant.

**STOMACH:** *(The stomach is associated with the color yellow, a sweet taste and the season of late summer.)*

The stomach is located in the upper abdomen between the esophagus and the small intestine. It is paired with the spleen. Located in the middle warmer, it represents the first big step in converting food into Qi. It receives food, stores and partially digests it and sends it on to the small intestine. It pushes down, while the spleen pushes up. The stomach is highly sensitive to emotion and is related to pensiveness or sympathy. If you are upset the stomach will not properly digest food and convert it into Qi and your whole system may potentially suffer.

**GALL BLADDER:** *(The gall bladder is linked with and affected by the emotion of anger and is associated with the color* *green, a sour taste, and the season of spring.)*

The gall bladder is paired with the liver and is located under its right lobe. The gall bladder stores and excretes the bile or gall produced by the liver. It helps control the health of muscles and joints. It also helps control the amount and quality of Qi in the system.

**URINARY BLADDER:** *(The bladder controls the emotion of fear and is associated with the color black, a salty taste and the season of winter.)*

The urinary bladder is located in the front part of the pelvic cavity. It is paired with the kidneys, one of the most important organs in Qigong, although the bladder itself has never been given the same amount of attention. Its main purpose is to transform fluid wastes into urine, hold them in its reservoir and then excrete them. Like the kidneys, it helps develop the brain, bones, and marrow.

## Healthy Organs and the Flow of Qi

This information on the meridians and internal organs is simply to help us realize what a wonderful body we have! Everything is designed to work together. If the yin and yang are balanced within us, we will be healthy, confident and effective in the world around us. This means maintaining the health of body, mind (including emotional states) and spirit.

In Qigong, we speak of the *three vitalities* or *three treasures* that must be considered and understood if we are to regulate body, mind and spirit. These are called *Jing, Qi* and *Shen*. They are inseparable and are aspects of the life energy.

The *Jing* comes from heredity and the food you eat. It affects biological functions, including the health of the blood, reproductive and endocrine systems. Jing is enhanced and maintained by taking care of the body, reducing stress, building and conserving your strength and energy, eating healthy food and practicing good habits.

The *Qi* is the vital force which energizes your total system. It is the *"electricity"* or energy that turns on and runs the "human machine." Qi energizes the Jing and Shen and without a healthy Qi supply the spiritual/mental/physical organism suffers. Breathing good air, eating correctly, practicing Qigong exercises and maintaining a positive attitude all enhance receptivity and integration of Qi.

*Shen* can be translated in many ways, but basically it means spirit or mind. Awareness of our higher spiritual nature depends upon our energy level, tranquility and mental stability. This is why in Qigong we practice breathing deeply, calming the mind, eliminating negativity, and nurturing confident, happy, peaceful and positive thoughts.

Good food, good air, good activity and good thoughts are all part of Qigong. All contribute to the nourishment and total well-being of our systems. We are reflections of our heredity, environment, and the daily choices we make for healthy living. We must continuously build, maintain and exchange our supply of Qi to live and experience a full and happy life.

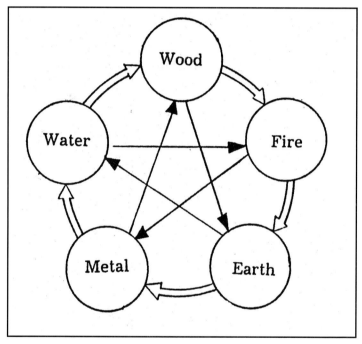

*Figure 3.9 The Five Elements*
*The five elements generate (empty arrows) and control (dark-pointed arrows) each other according to the above pattern. The elements also correspond with other aspects of existence. Refer to chart, page 46.*

Enlightenment

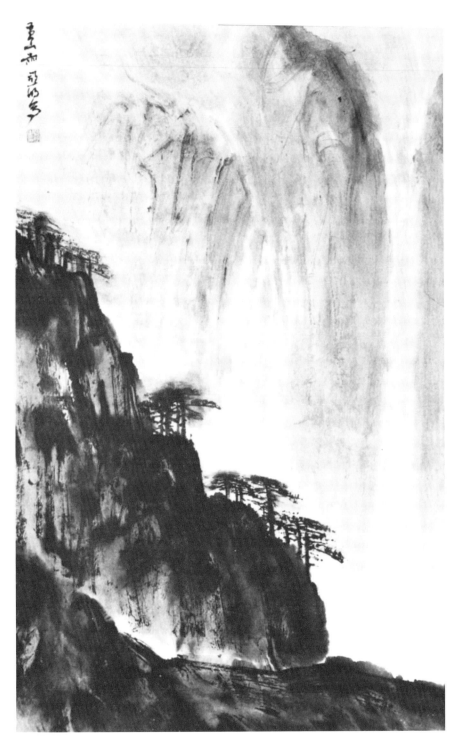

**Rain Huang-shan**
*(Yellow Mountain)*
Ya Ming (1924)

# CHAPTER 4

# BENEFITS OF QIGONG
# IN DAILY LIFE

*Paradise is where I am.*
–Voltaire –

## Wellspring of Health and Happiness

Benefits of Qigong are experienced in all aspects of life. By practicing this healing art program on a daily basis, you consistently develop Qi. Qigong is a self-therapy that releases blocked energy and allows it to flow smoothly through the meridians of the body. As a result, body, mind and spirit are brought into a harmonious state of being. Regardless of your interests and needs at the moment, Qigong will assist in developing greater clarity of mind and increased energy.

Through practicing The Eight Treasures, you learn to balance your own gift of energy.

Some of the overall benefits include:
1) Stress management
2) Developing a tremendous energy level
3) Mental focus, clarity and improved memory
4) Strengthened nervous and immune systems
5) Reduction or elimination of pain
6) Purification and rejuvenation of the whole body including internal organs, bones, circulation, skin, muscles
7) Elimination or decrease of various imbalances, allergies and/or diseases
8) Replacement of fear and anxiety with serenity, confidence and happiness
9) Enhancement of performance levels in school, work and sports

Scientific research on the therapeutic value of Qigong has been ongoing in China for many years, funded by the Chinese government. Modern hospitals or sanitariums, which focus on treating chronic diseases with Qigong, were established in China in the early 1950's. Qigong, of course, has been part of the traditional Chinese healing arts for thousands of years. Many more medical institutions today monitor and supervise the recovery of illness utilizing Qigong as a primary and/or supplementary treatment.

Most hospitals in China have Qigong units where patients learn self-healing practices and receive Qigong healing treatments. Qigong institutes throughout China not only do research, but train people to help themselves and others through the practice of these extraordinary exercises.

Although no scientific study has been able to identify the nature of Qi or even prove that it exists, the healing power of this force is well-documented. Studies on the benefits and qualities of internal Qi (inside the body) and external Qi (that which is emitted to others from a Qigong master or practitioner) are continuing. The emission of external Qi (healing energy) to others has been shown to have highly significant results in treating diseases. This has generated great scientific interest in many countries.

Several international conferences on Qigong have been held in Beijing, with China, the United States, Canada, Australia, Japan, European nations and other countries presenting current scientific findings on medical benefits of Qigong.

We know from ongoing research, for example, that Qigong practice increases alpha brain wave production in the frontal region of the brain. This could improve neural functions, regulate body processes and emotional imbalances. Increased alpha production is related to the Qigong mind state of "the thought of no thought." Increased alpha production also helps reduce stress, boost creative thinking and enhance mental clarity.

In addition, research has shown that Qigong also boosts the immune system by increasing the white blood cell count. This means that one is less susceptible to many diseases, allergies and other imbalances. Studies are ongoing today to ascertain and thus better understand if this is one reason Qigong practice is effective in treating certain cancers, and determining its effectiveness for helping people with the HIV virus or AIDS.

Research has also shown that Qigong improves circulation in all areas of the body, including an increase in the blood flow to nourish the brain. It helps lower high blood pressure and improves the health of the cardiovascular system.

Other research has indicated that Qigong regulates body metabolism, which includes endocrine function and improving secretion of digestive juices in the stomach and intestines. Practicing Qigong has helped many people regulate their weight, whether they needed to lose or gain.

Although *Chinese* medicine has associated emotional states with illness for thousands of years, it has been only recently that *Western* science is finding significant correlations between psychological make-up or personality patterns and certain diseases. We know that stress aggravates many conditions. Studies have shown that worry, anxiety, depression and negative thinking in general lower white blood cell count and leave the body more prone to blood disease.

Qigong emphasizes not only developing physical strength, health and energy, but maintaining a positive, calm, cheerful outlook in life.

It is no mystery that most of us want to be happy. How to achieve this is the big question. Happiness, of course, means many different things to different people. It might mean getting something you want, whether it is improved health, a good job, vacation, a marriage partner, new car, house – the list is endless. But through the ages the wisest among us have said that people and things external to yourself cannot give you happiness or guarantee peace of mind. You are the only one who can do that and it starts within.

This state of inner happiness is of the foremost importance in Qigong philosophy and training. A mind that is thinking happy thoughts and feeling confident is a mind that can nurture and direct the Qi. Every thought and emotion has its reaction or response in the body. Chinese philosophy does not see mind, body and spirit as separate. Everything is related to and a part of everything else.

A negative mind set impairs your total level of functioning – physically, mentally and spiritually. Negativity cuts you off from your spiritual source, your sustenance, the life force that pulses through your being.

Happiness comes from a mind or soul at peace with itself. This state of peace reflects inner harmony and balance. It is a feeling of wholeness. When the Qi is flowing smoothly and freely through the body, vitality is strong and you experience a natural feeling of optimism and joy. This is actually the state of harmony we are capable of experiencing day by day. But as the Chinese characters *Qi* and *gong* suggest, it takes daily practice to sustain this level of joyous, radiant and energized living.

Humankind's need to enjoy life has remained the same as centuries and cultures have come and gone. Continuous love and joy of life is directly related to several key ideas. First, the supply of Qi is inexhaustible. Second, we easily can learn how to tap into it, develop and direct it. Third, we are far greater than we have imagined. The source of the Tao is within the very heart of our being.

It's pretty simple, isn't it? The way to live a happy, healthy life is to cultivate your Qi, and indulge yourself in positive, loving thoughts and actions.

## Positive Personal Transformations

There are thousands of documented cases from people in all walks of life who have received tremendous help from Qigong practice and treatments. Very mild techniques are designed for those with severe illness. More moderate curative and preventative techniques, with which most people are familiar, are designed for daily well-being.

A self-therapeutic healing discipline, Qigong helps restore all areas of one's life. Some of the immediately obvious improvements are a feeling of deep serenity through managing stress more effectively. Through calming the mind, things that seemed upsetting and frustrating are seen with an expanded perspective. Meaningful solutions to problems often can be found.

In addition, the rejuvenation of the entire body, including internal body functions and structure, often results in disappearance or decrease of pain and problems that previously eluded traditional medical care.

The practice of releasing negative emotions has an

immediate boost on one's energy level and immune response. It also enhances overall creativity and insight.

The increased flow of Qi through the body also greatly enhances mental, physical and spiritual energy levels. It restores a feeling of radiance, lightness and buoyancy.

Students of Qigong have overcome major imbalances, diseases, pain and suffering in the course of their everyday lives. Complaints all but disappear: "*I had such a rough day. My neck hurts. I have a headache. Oh, my aching back.*"

The following are only a few of the many examples reported by students in The Eight Treasures of Qigong Program seminars and classes.

*No More Asthma:* A woman in her mid fifties had been suffering from terrible asthma attacks for a number of years. After only one Qigong session, she reported that she was free from her asthmatic condition. The symptoms have never returned.

Qigong has an excellent track record of helping or curing people with asthmatic symptoms. Acupuncture, also, has been proven highly effective in this area. Qigong is often called *acupuncture without needles* because it stimulates and utilizes the same energy meridians.

*The Vanishing Neck Pain:* A man in his thirties had suffered from such excruciating neck pain due to an injury which affected all areas of his life. Medical treatment and adjustments had been of no help. His wife was considering divorce. After practicing Qigong and opening the body to the flow of healing energy, his neck pain completely subsided. He was absolutely amazed and remained pain free. He returned to normal living and restored his marriage relationship.

*Beyond Menopausal Symptoms:* A woman in her mid fifties reported that since practicing Qigong she had not experienced any of the usual menopausal symptoms related to her age and change in life. She had no hot flashes, no depression, no fatigue. "I feel like I'm sixteen," she reported. "Qigong gives me the energy, harmony and balance I need to feel better than I ever have."

*Self-confidence Restored:* A young woman in her late twenties frequently felt intimidated at her job. One client in particular often called and made numerous demands, and she dreaded having to talk with him. She did not know how to respond to aggressive individuals. Whenever she was confronted by someone, she shrank into her shell.

After practicing Qigong for a few weeks she felt her self-confidence and mental clarity growing stronger and stronger. Soon she found herself handling the aggressive caller with diplomacy and firmness, and the problem melted away. She began to enjoy her interactions with all varieties of individuals, no longer being fearful of expressing herself or knowing the best course of action.

*Traumatic Pain Disappears:* A 60 year old man had spent over $10,000 for a week in the hospital. The doctors were trying to determine the cause and cure of multiple body aches and pains resulting from an accident. After no results he decided to try Qigong. Within only a few hours of gentle practice, he was freed from all pain and discomfort. He has continued to practice and the pain has not returned.

*Recognizing The Healing Energy:* After one practice session of Qigong a middle-aged nurse experienced tremendous heat in the lower Dan Tian. This healing energy spread throughout her body, increasing her energy level and well-being. She realized that this intensity of the healing force would greatly assist her in healing and administering to others.

*Quick Fix Of Rejuvenation:* A 55 year old executive reported that one afternoon he was so tired he planned to take a nap, yet there was quite a lot of work that needed to be done. Instead he began practicing Qigong for a few minutes, and immediately felt renewed. He abandoned his nap and continued with his reading and other work.

*Making A Life Transition:* An energetic woman in her fifties was generally happy with her job and life, and was not looking for anything special except to feel stronger and healthier. She began practicing Qigong, and soon experienced a new sense about herself and her life direction. A stronger, clearer vision began dawning in her consciousness.

She decided to leave her job and go back to school, making a career change and venturing into a whole new area. She attributed her sudden change of life direction to increased confidence and mental clarity.

*The End To Cold Feet:* A woman who had continuing problems with cold feet and poor circulation became aware of Qigong. Through practicing Qigong, the circulation in her feet greatly improved. Her feet became warm and remained at body temperature.

*The Reduction Of Tumors:* A man in his seventies began practicing Qigong when he was filled with malignant tumors. After receiving Qigong treatments, many of the tumors shrunk or disappeared. He recognized that his health depended upon the Qi flow to restore balance throughout his body.

*Instant Vacation:* A first time Qigong student arrived at the seminar highly stressed out. Daily life had become so difficult for her she had scheduled a vacation to Hawaii the following week, although she really didn't have the time to get away. After one session of practicing Qigong, she was completely renewed and relaxed. "I'm canceling my trip to Hawaii," she said, "I don't need it anymore." Her mind was clear, emotions calm, and spirit renewed. We can walk in paradise moment by moment if we know where to find it.

*Curing Daily Aches And Pains:* After moving heavy furniture around, a woman in her thirties had extremely tired and sore muscles. Although she felt like she barely could move, she practiced Qigong for a few minutes. The soreness and discomfort completely went away, and she was amazed that she could continue with setting up her new home.

*Giving Up The Victim Role:* A young married woman found herself the prime target of her husband's temper tantrums. She would shrink in the face of his anger and take the blame for his moods. Once she learned about Qigong, she developed her own inner sense of confidence and well-being. She was then able to maintain her strength and confront the situtation.

She was able to change from feeling victimized by another's anger to feeling empowered within herself. Her posture changed from slouching to upright and confident. She then proceeded to take positive steps through counseling to resolve their difficulties.

*Moving Through Difficult Times:* In the midst of a seemingly routine daily life, a 45 year old woman suddenly felt like everything was falling apart, including herself. She was diagnosed with cancer and her husband asked for a divorce.

During this traumatic time she discovered Qigong and began practicing on a daily basis. She explained that she soon developed a new inner calm, increased energy and feeling of well-being. She began the process of recovery and knew she was back in control of her life and her health once more.

*Overcoming Fear and Pain:* A middle-aged businessman decided to use his Qigong training when he had a benign growth surgically removed from his hand. He went to see his doctor and was administered a local anesthetic. He simply entered the state of mind he had learned through practicing Qigong – calm, relaxed and confident, with a sense of lightness and well-being. He was free from discomfort and fear and experienced a rapid, pain-free recovery.

*Miracle Session For Fibromyalgia:* After many trips to doctors and chiropractors with no results, a man suffering with fibromyalgia was desperate. This is a common ailment involving muscular and joint rheumatism and pain. He decided to try Qigong as a last resort, although he was skeptical and had canceled several appointments for private instruction.

When he showed up for a practice session, he was unable to move his neck and shoulders and couldn't extend his right arm. He gently practiced the first several postures and felt energy rushing through his body. All the debilitating pain in his body was washed away and he could freely move his neck, arms and shoulders. "This is a miracle", he exclaimed. "This is a wonderful self-treatment which has released all my pain. I can move again. If everyone would practice this, there would be nothing left for doctors!" He was thrilled with the results of his first Qigong session.

Students with diabetes, arthritis, heart disease, stroke and other ailments have been greatly helped through restoring their vital energy through Qigong practice. Women going through menopause often experience a reduction or disappearance of symptoms through Qigong training. Qigong offers a different gift to everyone, depending upon one's need, condition and orientation. The essence and reality of every gift is enhanced health and more joy in daily living.

# Qi's Healing Power

Everything thrives on energy. Everything *is* energy. Your body is alive because of the life force, or Qi, pulsing through it. The intake of food, water and air from the environment all are translated into energy for your system to use. Qi is our cosmic fuel. It is part of everything we experience.

Becoming more in tune with your body through Qigong practice, naturally creates a healthier, more nurturing lifestyle. As respect and love for yourself grow, you honor your being with healthy foods, loving thoughts and positive relationships. Maintaining balance in all areas of life becomes a priority.

There are untold benefits in all areas of life when we grasp the idea of self-reliance through self-care. Yet all too often people choose to disregard the rules of health and expect others to make them feel better. It takes only a few minutes to practice Qigong. It takes only a few moments to relax the mind and practice slow, calm, deep breathing. This stimulates many psychological and physical functions that contribute to healing and wholeness. No prescription is needed to take a deep breath and calm the mind. It is so simple and easy, yet we often forget the way of the Tao.

One of our greatest uses of Qi is directing its healing power to others. The benefits we derive from Qigong can be shared as we consciously emit healing energy to someone else through our mind and hands. Anyone can do this. We all participate in the same great energy flow and we are all a part of one another on a more expanded level of perception. Your power to promote the health and wholeness of loved ones, as well as yourself, will increase as you progress with your practice. (See "Healing Meditation", Chapter 8).

## The Tao of Doing and Being

An ancient Taoist saying is that the *Tao is ever inactive, yet there is nothing that it does not do.* The idea of *standing firmly on a moving point* has been the guideline for successful living in many philosophic disciplines. Basically, this means if our inner focus is calm and clear, open to receive the energy from the universe, all aspects of our lives will flow in health and harmony.

We act in the world based upon our perceptions. If our awareness is *being at one with the Tao*, then our *doing* or actions will be filled with positive intent and result in more favorable outcome. When we are filled with confidence, joy and happiness, life seems like "effortless effort." When times are difficult, we only need remember to open our minds to replenish our gift of energy from the universe. The whole world changes as we practice Qigong and fills to overflowing with the Tao every day.

*"When the mind is quiescent and void, true energy is at your command."*
The Yellow Emperor's Classic of Internal Medicine.

Tranquility

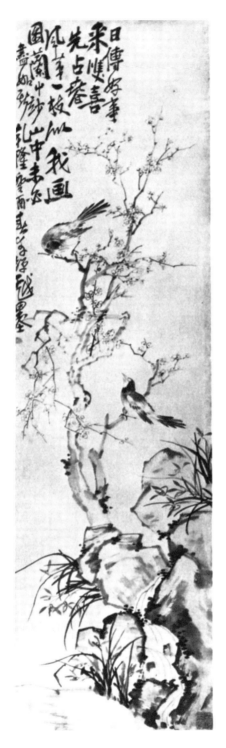

*Two Magpies, Plum Blossoms,*
*Orchids and Rocks*
Lu Shan  (1686-c. 1762)

# CHAPTER 5

# PRINCIPLES AND
# PRACTICE OF QIGONG

*Learning Qigong is like learning to ride a bicycle.*
*You can read all the books in the world about it, but*
*the only way to really learn is to practice doing it.*

## Three Keys to Practice

Many types of Qigong exercises have been developed over thousands of years and each school of thought has its own guidelines for practice. But three important factors have always remained the same: the mind, breathing and postures. Remembering these key ideas will enrich your experience, help you enjoy your practice more, hasten your understanding and bring greater benefits.

Just like the forces of yin and yang, they are part of one another and must be balanced to achieve maximum benefit from your Qigong practice. For example, the mind must be focused and relaxed to direct the Qi. Slow, calm breathing helps relax and open the mind and body to *receive the Qi energy*. It is important to remember that Qigong is about *receiving energy*, your gift from the universe. Movement combined with mental focusing and relaxation makes it easier to direct energy through the body.

## The Tranquil Mind

The mind is the greatest factor in developing your training. Calming the mind actually means calming *thoughts and emotions*. The emotions throw us into states of turmoil and interfere with our concentration. The brain needs a lot of energy to function well but, through stress and worry, we waste a great deal of it.

The wisdom mind is the higher intuitive voice that calmly guides us if we listen to it. It is part of our natural awareness that is always present and reliable.

Learning to maintain a calm, still mind in the midst of motion is part of Qigong training. Slow, focused movements heighten awareness. A tranquil mind doesn't mean being spaced out or half asleep. It means being relaxed yet alert, peaceful yet aware, flowing gently in harmony with breathing and movements.

In Chinese medicine we believe that almost all illness is the result of emotional imbalances. That is why we talk so much about the importance of cultivating positive emotions and releasing negative thoughts and feelings. This negativity is mental garbage and disrupts the flow of Qi in your system. A tranquil state creates the positive effect of protecting your organism and health.

Take a moment to do a little experiment. First, recall a time when you were feeling unsure of yourself, embarrassed or self-conscious. Deliberately remember the emotions you experienced. It may have been several years ago or minutes ago. Just be aware of those feelings and see what they do to your body and mind. Fear, depression, anxiety, self-doubt or any negative feelings cause your energy to drop and dull mental functioning. They block the flow of Qi.

Second, remember a time when you felt especially confident and were enjoying yourself. Things were going well. This may be any time, past or present, as long as the memory is clear. You will feel a definite shift in your mental and physical energy. Just recalling a happy, confident time increases energy, the Qi flow in mind and body and builds resistance to disease!

How powerful is the mind! That is why deliberately cultivating tranquility, a cheerful mood, confidence, happiness and respect for self and others is so critical to overall well-being. Mental energy can be preserved if the mind is calm.

Not only does the quality of your emotions affect your own mind and body, but other people are influenced by your emotional states. Perhaps you have heard the story of the man who goes to work and is yelled at by his boss. He comes home and yells at his wife. She gets upset, yells at her son, then he goes outside and vents his anger on the dog!

Developing a Qigong mind means being aware and in control of emotional states. One must avoid sacrificing health and happiness through negativity. Through practicing Qigong breathing and focusing exercises, you soon will be integrating more positive emotions and confident actions into everyday life.

## Breathing Techniques

There are many methods of Qigong breathing, and each accomplishes a slightly different purpose. Whatever form you use, remember it should be slow, calm, deep and smooth. The four techniques discussed below are commonly used in Qigong training. The first method, natural breathing, is recommended for the exercises in The Eight Treasures Program. Your own breathing will develop naturally as you progress with Qigong practice.

*1. Natural Breathing:* This is your current pattern of breathing. To regulate natural breathing means simply to focus the mind on your pattern of breathing and make it slower, smoother, deeper, calmer and quieter. This works much better than trying a different method of breathing that you are not used to doing. In addition to following your natural breathing pattern, try to remember to inhale through the nose and exhale through the mouth. While doing the postures it is important to feel relaxed and comfortable.

*2. Abdominal Breathing:* In this method, breathe all the

way down to the Dan Tian center below the navel. When inhaling, expand the abdomen and when exhaling contract it. This is done in the lower abdomen, so do not expand and contract the chest. Do not hold your breath. This is often called breathing like a child, because it is the natural and easy breathing of most children. This constant back and forth movement massages the internal organs and stimulates abdominal muscles.

*3. Reverse Abdominal Breathing:* This method is used by Taoist practitioners and is often called Taoist breathing. When inhaling, contract the abdomen and when exhaling, expand the abdomen. This has the same health benefits as abdominal breathing and, in addition, serves to conserve and direct Qi into the body's extremities.

*4. Chest Breathing:* This involves expanding the chest or rib cage when inhaling, contracting the chest or rib cage when exhaling. This method increases the capacity of the lungs and is often used by those in the external martial arts or in such areas as weight lifting and deep sea diving. It is also a technique employed in Yoga because it increases the oxygen supply throughout the body. It is important to be relaxed when doing this breathing method.

It may take a little practice to really get the feel of breath coordination, but soon the body's inhalations and exhalations will flow easily with your movements and postures.

Before beginning Qigong, breathe naturally a few times and let your mind relax. While inhaling, direct the breath energy down through the lungs to the lower Dan Tian, the internal area several inches below the navel. Imagine the breath energy flowing into the Dan Tian, picturing it as light energy if you wish. Using this area as the main focus of concentration during Qigong practice centers your mind and develops your energy.

Slow, rhythmic deep breathing helps balance the yin and yang energy within and around your being. It drives this energy throughout all the body's meridians and spreads into the energy field encircling the body, creating a protective, radiant Qi shield around you.

Natural, slow, calm, smooth deep breathing is recommended for The Eight Treasures. With persistance, patience and practice, the program will enable you to develop concentration and guide the energy through your body.

## Postures

Each posture or movement is done smoothly, slowly, and calmly to the individual's comfort level. It provides a framework through which energy flows. In Qigong there is inward and outward motion. Mental energy or thought is integrated with rhythmic physical action. One always moves with awareness. Qigong has been called meditation in motion, which means that mental focusing is integrated with movement. This is the easiest way to guide the Qi.

The principle behind doing the postures is entirely different from regular exercise in which you tax the muscles. Here, strength and vitality are developed through the flowing of Qi energy, not through physical stress on the body.

Every movement and every posture integrates, exchanges and balances the yin and yang, working with internal energy, external energy or both. Your internal energy is the same as universal energy. When the forces of body, mind and spirit are in harmony with the Tao, your life unfolds in a healthy, balanced way.

Also, there are several guidelines to keep in mind when doing the postures which may help promote a better energy flow:

a) *Hand placement.* When the posture suggests that hands be placed together in front of the body, one behind the other, the male places the left hand behind the right hand; and the female places the right hand behind the left. This hand placement helps balance the dominant yang energy in males and the dominant yin energy in females.

b) *Tongue placement.* During practice, the tip of the tongue may be placed gently on the middle of the upper hard palate. This is just a light touch, not a push. This point at the roof of the mouth and the tip of the tongue connects the two major channels which circulate through the body: the Conception Channel in front and the Governing Channel in back. The tongue serves as a link in the energy flow.

The simple yet elegant postures presented here are

always done in a relaxed manner: slowly, smoothly and naturally. There are no exact positions, no correct or incorrect ways to do them. Rather, they are done to each person's needs, individuality and comfort.

This is easy to understand when we realize, once again, that hundreds of variations of any one posture might exist, depending upon the guidance of individual masters and schools of Qigong. A posture simply provides an expanded medium in your body for the flowing of Qi, a variation of focus and direction of energy. The goal is always the same: to establish an overall supply and balance of Qi within your total system to promote health and well-being.

## Focus and Visualization

All of the Qigong exercises in the preparation, The Eight Treasures and meditations involve focusing, sensing and visualization. The ability to focus or concentrate is the ability to direct your mental energy at will, or to center your mind. Gently guiding, sensing and/or visualizing your mental energy during the Qigong exercises greatly increases your concentration ability.

For example, in the first preparation exercise, you are asked to imagine you are collecting energy from the earth and bringing it into your body. To do this it is helpful to picture yourself standing in a beautiful garden, collecting energy from vibrant trees, bright green grass, blooming fragrant flowers and whatever beautiful plants you wish to envision. You are also asked to imagine you are collecting energy from deep within the earth. This has a centering, grounding effect, and you will begin to feel the flow of energy in your hands and feet.

Remember that thoughts direct energy, and visualization is a thought picture. Thought pictures are extraordinarily useful tools in guiding Qi and gaining control of your energy and health. Relaxed focusing on these thought images increases their power.

## Avoiding the Perfection Trap

In many sports and competitive activities, the emphasis is on doing it better than someone else, doing it right, pushing to the point of pain to create stronger muscles, studying harder to learn more facts and figures. These involve struggle and effort in trying to perform a certain way, look a certain way, be a certain way. The emphasis is on getting it right, winning and being the best in your field.

This notion of perfection seeps into all aspects of our thinking, whether its about physical beauty, skill, performance, knowledge, or even taking the right kinds of vitamins and eating the right kinds of food.

Qigong exercises recognize and emphasize the need and comfort level for each individual. There is no straining, just gentle movement. The exercises should feel effortless and flowing. Directing the Qi with the mind is likewise done in a gentle, relaxed way. Simply move your awareness to the various areas of the body. This is not really difficult. If you hurt your hand, all of your attention goes to the hand. If you have an itch on your back or shoulder, the attention moves to the specific area. Directing attention to a specific area, moving it up and down the body, is the way in which you direct and build Qi. The Qi energy is already flowing through meridians and vessels, and your mindful focusing enables it to flow in a better and stronger way.

So when you are doing the postures, imagine you are directing Qi energy throughout the body. Imagine that it is gently, evenly and increasingly flowing to various areas, whether to the top of the head, legs and feet, arms and hands, or throughout your internal organs. You soon will be able to experience the movement of energy throughout the body by becoming aware of it, tuning into it with your mind.

Remember that one of the mental reference points for successful Qigong practice is self respect and respect for others. The more you honor and respect yourself the more you will be aware of your energy and needs. Honor your individuality, relax and follow the general guidelines. This is the basis for successful practice.

## Why Preparation Exercises?

The preparation exercises presented in Chapter Six are an integral part of the Qigong program. The suggested visualization and movement in each preparation exercise provide a framework for opening yourself to the infinite energy of the universe, the unseen life force, and establishing mental and physical harmony with this energy.

This experience of harmony or balance produces a tranquil mind set which promotes the flow of Qi throughout your being. During the preparation time you are building your reservoir of Qi. Then, when practicing The Eight Treasures you will realize even greater benefit and will more readily experience the energy flow in your body.

You might think of them as warm-up movements, just as you would do gentle stretching and bending before engaging in more vigorous exercise. The Eight Treasures look simple to do, and they are, but you are working with powerful channels of energy in your body. A little preparation will heighten awareness, receptivity and beneficial results.

## Practicing Qigong

Some say you should not practice Qigong after a meal, when tired or sleepy, or when under a lot of stress with too many things on your mind. Some say practice at the same time every day to sensitize the body to receiving an increase of Qi at regular intervals. All this counsel has merit, of course, but if we waited for ideal conditions many of us would never practice at all!

Practice whenever, wherever and whatever time you can. If you are tired, the movements and breathing exercises will help rejuvenate your body and mind. If you are worried and stressed out, collecting energy in the Preparation exercises will help renew and center you.

Just remember that you do need to practice to receive benefit so it is important to schedule these gentle exercises into your day.

## Summary

Remember that the mind is very powerful. A Qigong mind is tranquil and calm. Breathing, regardless of the posture or movement, is always slow, deep, smooth and quiet, not shallow or jerky. The postures are always done with flowing, even, comfortable movements. Each individual is different and no two people move in the exact same way. If something is uncomfortable, modify it to suit you.

Regardless of the suggested number of times to perform each posture or movement, remember your comfort level. Even if you can do only a few, then that's what you follow. Do not strain or struggle. Soon the movements should feel effortless.

When practicing Qigong, allow the mind to become very quiet. Practice Qigong confidently and with great respect toward other people and yourself. All you need to think about is what you are doing. As the energy flows through you, allow nature to take its course. It will instinctively guide you and the energy will do what it does best; heal, balance and energize.

The results will be positive, loving and unique to you. Tranquillity will result as one of your immediate benefits. Enjoy your body and mind. The more peaceful you feel, the happier and healthier you will be!

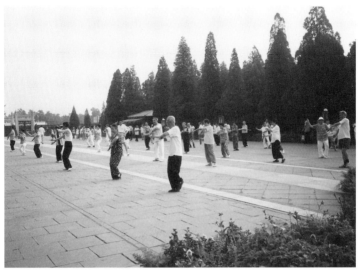

*Figure 5.0: Group practice in Beijing, China. It is a common occurrence in Beijing and other cities in China to hold public exercise sessions of Qigong in the early morning hours each day. One can simply stop and join in for as long as one wishes, no fee required.*

*Figure 5.1: Ms. Ballin participating in a public Qigong practice in China.*

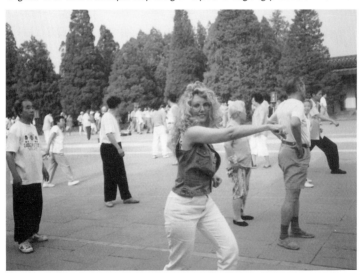

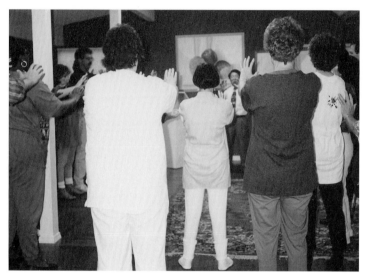

*Figure 5.2: Dr. Deng teaching The Eight Treasures to students in Houston, Texas. Fall, 1996.*

*Figure 5.3: Dr. Deng and students in The Eight Treasures workshop presented at The Plaza Hotel, New York, Summer 1997.*

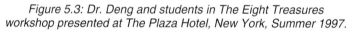

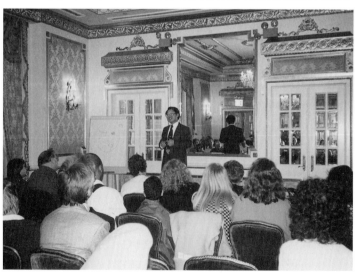

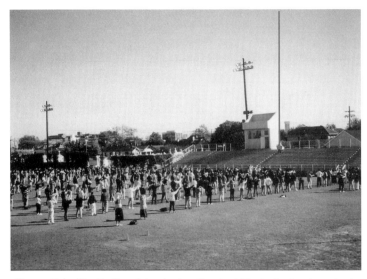

*Figure 5.4: Ms. Ballin giving instruction to 400 students at a private school in New Orleans, 1995: Collecting energy from the sun.*

*Figure 5.5: Dr. Deng answering questions during a Qigong seminar in Alaska, 1996.*

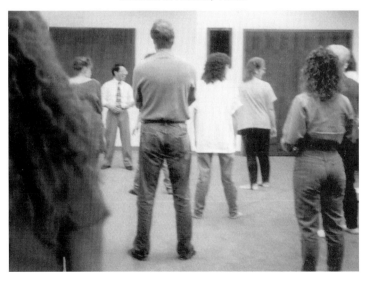

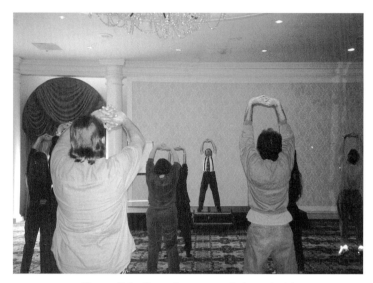

*Figure 5.6: One of many workshops held
in New Orleans, Louisiana.*

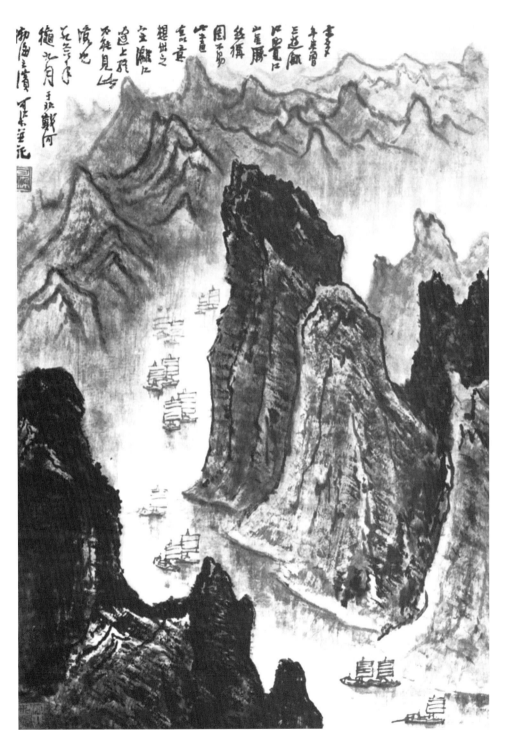

*Landscape,* 1966
Li K'o-jan (b.1907)

# CHAPTER 6

# BASIC PREPARATION FOR THE EIGHT TREASURES

*Opening your mind and body to the flow of the*
*Unseen Life Force revitalizes your health.*

## Beginning the Preparation

These five preparation exercises are an integral part of your Qigong program and are performed prior to the Treasures. They quiet your mind, focus awareness, open your energy and build the Qi.

You are opening your mind to the Tao, the universal life force, harmonizing internal and external energy. The collecting or gathering of energy represents bringing into balance your internal yin and yang forces with the external yin and yang energies.

For example, you begin by collecting energy from the

*earth*, which means opening yourself to the flow of predominantly yin energy. Then you collect energy from the *sun*, which is predominantly yang energy. Third, you go to the *ocean*, which is back to yin. Fourth, you collect energy from the *sky*, which is primarily yang.

In the fifth preparation movement you collect energy from the *whole universe*, which suggests opening mind, body and spirit to the flow of the Tao. This represents the perfect balance of yin and yang, externally and internally, your own being in harmony with the universal forces.

You may feel subtle shifts in your experience of energy when moving from one preparation posture to the next. This is because you are shifting between yin and yang energy forces. However, don't look for qualitative shifts or changes in your experience. *Enjoy* the visualizations, movements and collecting the energy. Your experience will be unique, exactly what it should be.

Although most movements are recommended eight times each, they may be performed in any number depending upon personal need. You may also perform the movements individually, while sitting, standing or reclining, adapting them to your requirements. It is best to wear comfortable clothes.

All the preparation postures are done with relaxed, slow, smooth movements, eyes lightly closed to assist in visualization. Each preparation movement flows into the next.

Breathing is natural, quiet, smooth and slow, and is coordinated with the movements. It is suggested that you inhale through the nose, and exhale through the mouth. Touch the tip of your tongue to the roof of your mouth.

To begin the following preparation phase, stand comfortably, with your feet parallel or placed to your comfort level, shoulder-width apart. Relax your arms by your sides. (Fig. 6.0) Let your whole body relax. Take three deep breaths, and lightly close your eyes.

*It is important to remember that Qigong is about receiving energy – your gift from the universe.*

The more harmonious and tranquil you feel, the healthier you are. The quieter your mind, the more you are aware of the Qi.

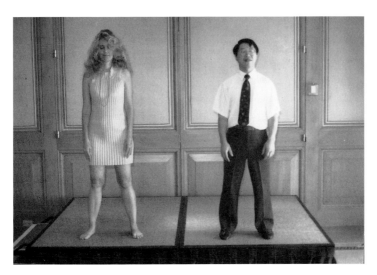

*Figure 6.0: Relaxed standing posture for beginning the preparation movements in The Eight Treasures of Qigong.*

# 1. Collecting Energy from the Earth

*Focus:* Mentally picture yourself standing in a beautiful garden, gathering energy from all around you. Imagine you are drawing energy into your body and mind from vibrant green trees, emerald grass, and fragrant blooming flowers. Also, imagine you are collecting energy from deep within the earth, and that this energy is flowing into your being.

You might experience energy in your hands or feet, particularly that it is flowing into your hands. You may feel various sensations in your palms, such as, heat, density, or tingling.

*Movement:* Extend both arms to the front, palms facing downward, and then raise your arms approximately to your shoulder level, or waist level if it is more comfortable. (Fig. 6.1). Then slightly lower your arms, and gently bend your knees. (Fig. 6.2) Again, raise the arms back to your shoulder height, and imagine you are drawing energy up from the earth and the beautiful garden, filling your body.

Inhale while raising the arms, and exhale while lowering the arms. Continue this gentle up and down movement with your arms, coordinated with your breathing, eight times.

*It is so easy to experience the life force. Focus your mind, breathe deeply and slowly, move gently and freely.*

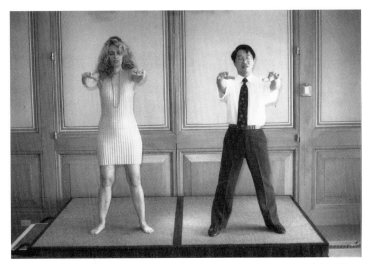

*Figure 6.1: Beginning posture for collecting EARTH ENERGY.*

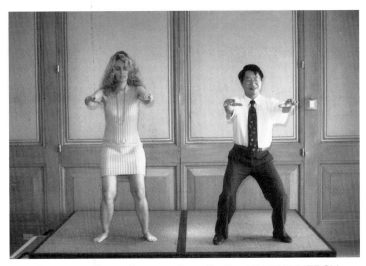

*Figure 6.2: Second posture for collecting EARTH ENERGY.*

## 2. Collecting Energy From the Sun

*Focus:* Mentally picture yourself standing on a mountain watching a sunrise or sunset. Imagine collecting radiant energy from the sunshine, drawing it into your mind and body with your arms and hands. Imagine this light energy filling your being.

You might experience warmth on your face, warmth or energy in your hands, feet or anywhere in your body. Just relax and enjoy whatever you experience. It is all the Qi.

*Movement:* Fully extend both arms in front of your body toward your mental image of the sun (Fig. 6.3). Bend the elbows, moving the hands towards the neck area, bringing the energy into your head, neck and face. (Fig. 6.4)

Inhale when bringing your arms and the sun energy toward your body and exhale when extending your arms toward the sun. Repeat this gentle movement, coordinated with your breathing, eight times.

*Develop a Qigong mind. Respect your mind enough to give it a healthy diet of positive thoughts, day after day.*

*As you practice Qigong you allow confidence, happiness and peace of mind to flow into your everyday life.*

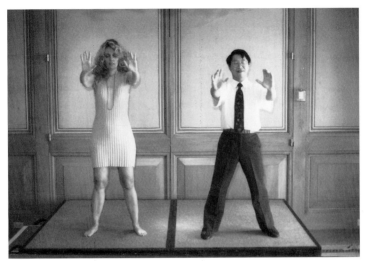

*Figure 6.3: Beginning posture for collecting SUN ENERGY.*

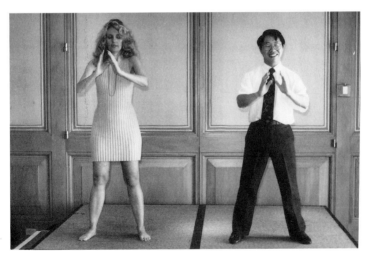

*Figure 6.4: Second movement for collecting SUN ENERGY.*

## 3. Collecting Energy from the Ocean

*Focus:* Mentally picture yourself standing on a vast shoreline surrounded by the water. Envision yourself collecting energy from the depths of this mighty ocean, from the rolling waves and the rhythm of the tides. Bring the energy of the ocean into your body, mind and spirit.

Be mindful of these wonderful feelings of filling yourself with the powerful energy of the ocean.

*Movement:* Extend your arms out to your sides at approximately shoulder level (Fig. 6.5). Turn your head to the right, imagining you are collecting energy with your hands from an endless stretch of this mighty ocean. Now turn your head forward again as you return your arms, elbows gently bent, to extend in front of you at shoulder level (Fig. 6.6). Repeat this process again turning toward the left side.

Alternate turning the head to the left and right sides, inhaling when you are gathering energy with your arms open, and exhaling when you return to the center. Repeat this process, coordinated with your breathing, eight times.

*The old phrase, "Use it or lose it" is especially applicable to Qigong. Develop and use the Qi consistently and you will maintain and enjoy vitality and longevity.*

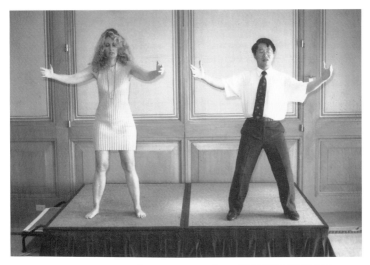

*Figure 6.5: Extending arms to collect OCEAN ENERGY.*

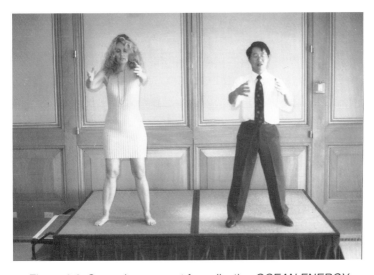

*Figure 6.6: Second movement for collecting OCEAN ENERGY.*

# 4. Collecting Energy from the Sky

*Focus:* Mentally picture yourself standing on a quiet mountainside, gazing into the night sky. Imagine gathering energy from the sky, from the stars, and from the new moon as it rises in the heavens. (Visualize a new moon, not a full moon or waning moon. The new moon represents the beginning of a new phase and increased energy.)

*Movement:* Begin with arms in front of your body, elbows gently bent, and your hands placed a few inches in front of the lower Dan Tian area. (Fig. 6.7) Bring the arms up in front of your body and extend them above your head, collecting energy from the sky. (Fig. 6.8) Then making a complete circle with your outstretched arms, bring them around to your sides and return the hands to the lower Dan Tian area.

Inhale when reaching your arms up to the sky and collecting energy, and exhale when returning the arms in a circle to your sides. Repeat this process eight times, coordinated with your breathing.

*The Tao is the eternal law at work in the universe. It is the principle behind all change. The world of being emerges from the interplay of yin and yang. What does this mean? Find harmony in your life.*

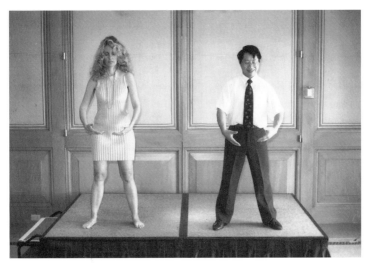

*Figure 6.7: Beginning posture for collecting SKY ENERGY.*

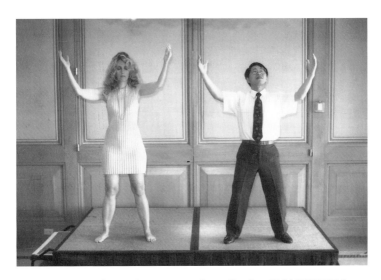

*Figure 6.8: Second movement for collecting SKY ENERGY.*

## 5. Collecting Energy from the Universe

*Focus:* Imagine gazing up into the infinite heavens, gathering energy from the whole universe, letting it flow into your being.

*Movement:* This is one continuous movement from the end of "sky energy". (Fig. 6.7) Begin inhaling at lower Dan Tian area. Bring your arms up in front of your body, palms facing each other toward an upward direction. (Fig. 6.9) Slowly extend the arms above your head. Forming a half circle with your outstretched arms, move them to shoulder level. (Fig. 6.10)

You are looking up into the universe, arms outstretched, gathering the universal energy, or Qi. Now exhaling, reverse the direction of movement, returning the arms over your head, back down in front of your body with the palms facing each other, fingertips pointing upward. Imagine you are depositing all the Qi in your lower Dan Tian, about three inches below the navel.

Inhale while reaching the arms to the sky and stretching them out at the shoulder level; exhale when returning the arms and placing hands on the Dan Tian. Practice this movement one time. Take three deep breaths. You are ready to begin the First Treasure.

*One who knows others is wise; one who knows the self is enlightened. – Lao-Tzu*

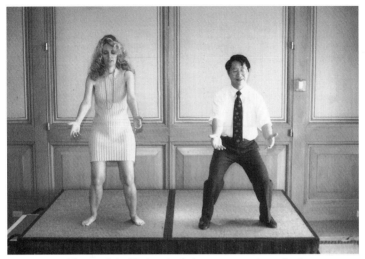

*Figure 6.9:  To begin, bring arms up to collect
energy from the UNIVERSE.*

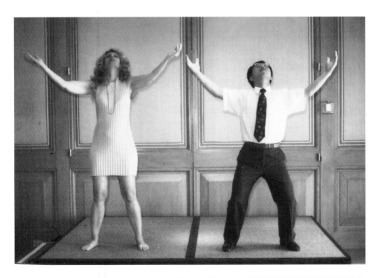

*Figure 6.10: Second movement for collecting UNIVERSE ENERGY.*

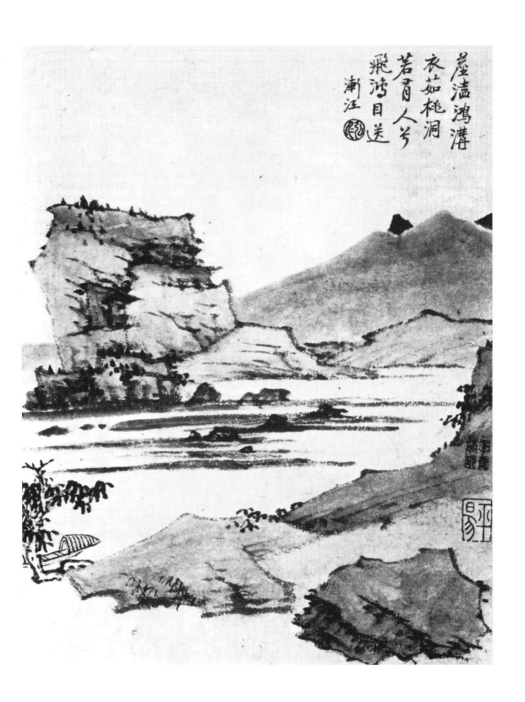

滄溘鴻漙
衣茹桃洞
若肯人兮
飛鴻目送
漸江 [印]

*Craggy Rocks and Watery Flatlands*
Hung Jen  (1610-1664)

# CHAPTER 7

# THE EIGHT TREASURES

*Be calm, silent and sincere in your daily practice*
*of these Treasures and you will unlock their*
*gifts of inner balance, health*
*and deep serenity.*

In this program there are The Eight Fundamental Treasures, with about eight movements for each treasure. This is traditional, classic, organized Qigong. A treasure is something of great value, a cherished prize or resource. As you perform each treasure, it reveals to you the revitalizing power of Qi, the gift of your own inner wealth and health.

Regular practice of these movements will guide you to cherish and nurture your own being. You will begin to enjoy greater energy, deep serenity, improved health, mental clarity and higher awareness.

## Beginning The Treasures

The Eight Treasures begin after the completion of the preparation exercises. You have relaxed mind and body, gathered energy and have taken three deep breaths after collecting energy from the universe. Lightly close your eyes.

# TREASURE #1:
## Developing the Triple Warmer

*Focus:* In the First Treasure, you develop your internal energy and direct it through the triple warmer. The triple warmer includes major energy reservoirs located in the lower, middle and upper Dan Tian regions.

The lower Dan Tian, about three inches below the navel and two inches inside includes the kidneys, small intestine, large intestine and bladder. The middle Dan Tian, located in the solar plexus area, includes the spleen, liver and stomach. The upper Dan Tian, located in the upper chest, includes the lungs, heart and brain. In this exercise you are guiding the energy with your mind, bringing it up through the triple warmer, letting it flow into your arms and hands as you reach over your head, raising heels slightly off the ground as you extend upward. Touch the sky with your hands, then bring the energy back to the lower Dan Tian, lowering the heels as you do so.

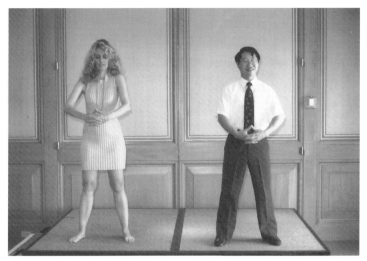

*Figure 7.0: Beginning posture for TREASURE 1*

***Posture:*** Stand with feet parallel or placed to comfort level, shoulder-width apart, and let your whole body relax. Interlock fingers and place your hands a few inches in front of and facing the lower Dan Tian at the navel. (Fig. 7.0)

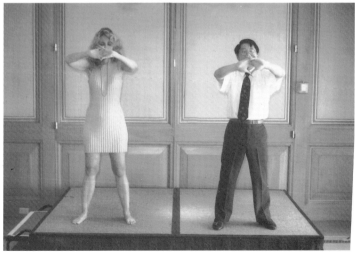

*Figure 7.1: Rotating palms. TREASURE 1.*

*Movement:* Take a deep breath and relax. Feel or imagine the Qi energy in the lower Dan Tian, then slowly raise your arms, moving the energy up through the triple warmer. When you reach the neck area, rotate your interlocked hands, palms facing outward. (Fig. 7.1) Continue to gently extend the arms above your head with the palms facing upward. Sustain position for a few seconds, lifting up your heels to lightly touch the sky with your hands. Don't send energy. (Fig. 7.2) Then lower the heels.

Keeping fingers interlocked and palms facing outward, return arms and hands to the original position.

Inhale when you begin, moving the energy up through the triple warmer. Begin exhaling when you reach neck area and exhale completely when touching the sky. Gently hold the breath when you return to the original position, moving the energy back to the Dan Tian. Complete movement eight times.

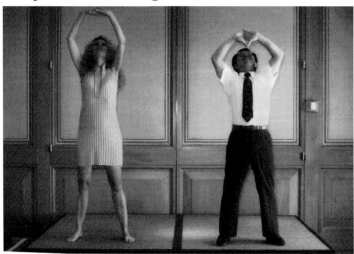

*Figure 7.2: Touching the sky. TREASURE 1.*

# TREASURE #2:
## Drawing the Bow and Arrow

*Focus:* In the Second Treasure you are working with both internal and external energy. You build internal energy and send it out to the universe. In this exercise, you move the Qi from the lower Dan Tian, through the triple warmer and send it out through your shoulders, arms and fingers. Imagine drawing a bow, shooting an arrow into a target.

*Posture:* The starting position is called the Horse Stance. Place your feet about two and one half foot lengths apart, a little wider than your shoulders, and bend the knees. Place your hands together a few inches in front of the lower Dan Tian. (A woman places her right hand inside the left hand, and a man places his left hand inside the right.) (Fig. 7.3).

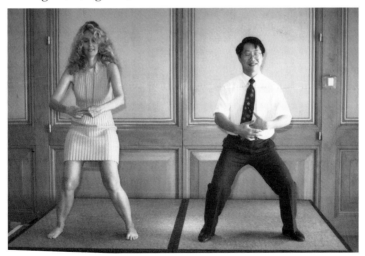

*Figure 7.3: The Horse Stance. TREASURE 2.*

*Movement:* Take a deep breath and relax. Move your hands from the lower Dan Tian, directing energy through shoulders, arms and hands.

Imagine you are going to shoot a bow and arrow toward the right. Fully extend the right hand to the right side, with middle and index fingers pointing out on both hands. Keep your left hand at about the waist level, the left elbow bent, the left hand also pointing toward the right. Pull and release an imaginary bow (Fig. 7.4). (You are releasing energy through your hands which can be directed toward others and used for healing.)

Alternate to the left (Fig. 7.5) and right sides. Inhale while moving the energy into your arms and hands, exhale while pulling and releasing the bow, and gently hold the breath when returning hands to the lower Dan Tian.

Complete this movement eight times.

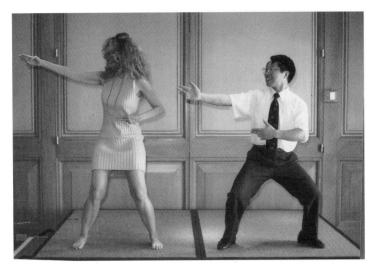

*Figure 7.4: Drawing the bow and arrow, right. TREASURE 2.*

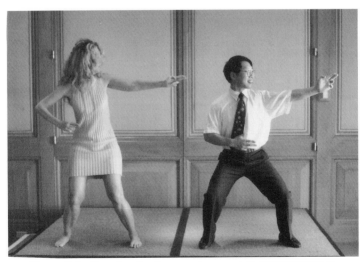

*Figure 7.5: Drawing the bow and arrow, left. TREASURE 2.*

# TREASURE #3:
## Balancing the Yin and Yang

*Focus:* In the Third Treasure you are again working with internal energy, balancing the yin and yang. You are not sending energy out into the universe, just touching the external energy field with the internal yin and yang forces. We all need a dynamic balance of yin and yang energy within ourselves to maintain health and strength.

In this Treasure you bring energy up from the lower Dan Tian, through the triple warmer, sending energy to both arms and hands; one reaching down to touch the earth and the other reaching up to touch the sky. The upper hand is yang energy, representing high, bright, hot sunshine (masculine, positive, external); the lower hand is yin energy, representing the deep, dark, cold earth (feminine, negative, internal).

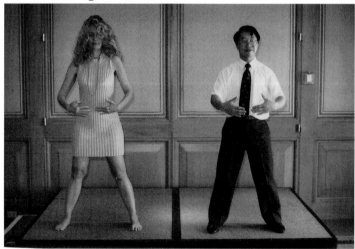

*Figure 7.6: Beginning hand movement. TREASURE 3.*

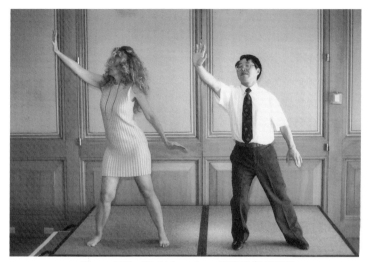

*Figure 7.7: Right hand up. TREASURE 3.*

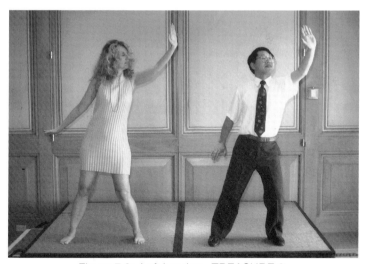

*Figure 7.8: Left hand up. TREASURE 3.*

113

*Posture:* Stand with feet parallel or placed to your comfort level, shoulder-width apart, and let your whole body relax. Relax your arms and place your hands together, palms inward, a few inches in front of the lower Dan Tian.

(A woman places her right hand inside the left hand and a man places his left hand inside the right.)

*Movement:* Take a deep breath and relax. Move your hands from the lower Dan Tian (Fig. 7.6), directing energy into your arms and hands. Reach down and out to the left side with the left arm, palm facing down, and up and out to the right side with the right arm, palm facing up.

The head turns toward the yin (lower) arm position first, then gradually turns up toward the yang (higher) arm position. (Fig. 7.7) Then, return the hands to the Dan Tian area.

Alternate sides, with the right arm reaching down (Fig. 7.8) and the left arm reaching up.

Inhale as you move your arms into position and exhale at full arm extension. Gently hold the breath when returning the hands to the lower Dan Tian.

Complete this movement eight times.

# TREASURE #4:
## Awakening the Third Eye

*Focus:* In the Fourth Treasure you are developing your third eye energy. The third eye area is located between the eyebrow and extends to the front and top of your head as you develop it. This is an important center for stimulating your brain and opening your psychic or intuitive perception. It also helps you learn to direct Qi energy like a laser beam throughout your body. This is especially helpful for self-empowerment and effectiveness in healing.

This exercise develops internal energy and works with the body's energy field. You move energy with your mind from the lower Dan Tian, through the triple warmer and direct it to the third eye area on the forehead between the eyebrows.

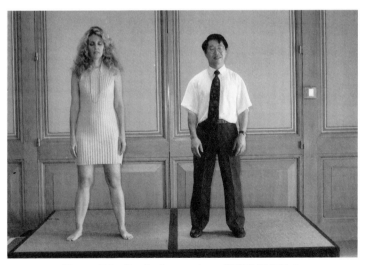

*Figure 7.9: Beginning posture. TREASURE 4.*

*Posture:* Stand with feet parallel or placed to your comfort level, shoulder-width apart. Let your body relax. Your arms rest gently at your sides (Fig. 7.9)

*Movement:* Take a deep breath and relax. Inhale as you move the Qi with your mind from the lower Dan Tian, through the triple warmer, to the third eye. (Imagine the energy moving up your body to your forehead.) Concentrate on the third eye area. Turn your head back over your right shoulder, and open your eyes to glance at your left heel. Exhale while shooting energy with the third eye to the left heel. (Fig. 7.10) Close your eyes again as you slowly turn to face forward. Gently holding the breath, draw energy with your mind up from the left heel through the inner left leg (liver meridians). Deposit the energy back into the lower Dan Tian.

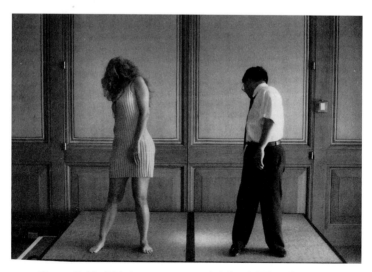

Figure 7.10: *Third eye energy to left heel. TREASURE 4.*

116

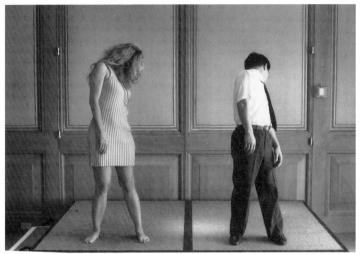

*Figure 7.11: Third eye energy to right heel, front view TREASURE 4.*

Alternate sides. Bring energy to the third eye, looking over left shoulder. Glance at the right heel while shooting energy to it with the third eye (Figs. 7.11 and 7.12, front and back views). Close your eyes as you bring energy back up from the inner right leg to the Dan Tian.

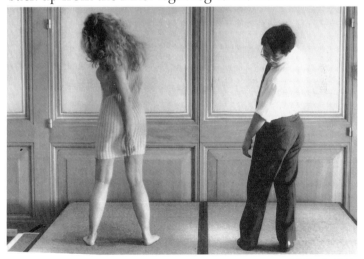

*Figure 7.12: Third eye energy to right heel, back view. TREASURE 4.*

You may wish to imagine the energy as a stream of light projected out from the third eye which you then move through your body.

Inhale when pulling the energy up through body. Exhale when directing it through the third eye. Gently hold breath when returning to deposit the energy in the Dan Tian. Complete movement eight times.

# TREASURE #5:
## Eliminating Negative Emotions

*Focus:* In the Fifth Treasure it is important to concentrate fully on the Qi in the lower Dan Tian, internally about two to three inches below the navel. You are working with internal energy, clearing the mind and releasing negative emotions and feelings.

You are throwing away the garbage in your mind: anger, anxiety, irritability, fear, crabbiness, hostility, inferiority – the list might be quite extensive. All negativity is being released during this Treasure.

By learning to rest the mind in the lower Dan Tian, you begin to understand that you do not have to identify with existing negative thought patterns. As you balance your energy and develop your breathing patterns, you feel healthier and stronger. You gain a calmer, happier, more positive outlook and achieve harmony and balance automatically. Negative emotions will begin to flow away and return your heart and mind to its original state of love and peace.

*Posture:* Stand relaxed in the Horse Stance position, with feet about two and one half foot lengths apart, wider than your shoulders, and bend knees. Place your hands on your thighs, thumbs pointing backward, to achieve a solid, balanced footing. (Fig. 7.13)

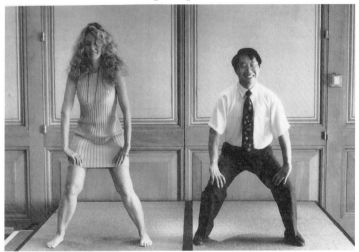

*Figure 7.13: Beginning posture for TREASURE 5.*

*Movement:* Take a deep breath. As you exhale imagine releasing all negative thoughts and emotions. Relax. Gently rotate your neck and head in a clockwise direction, doing neck rolls, making small circles. Inhale when rolling head down and forward (Fig. 7.14). Exhale when rolling the head around and back. (Fig. 7.15) Repeat four times clockwise, and four times counterclockwise, making a set of eight.

Repeat the same rotations making larger circles with your whole upper body. (Fig. 7.16) Allow body to move naturally and loosely. Inhale when moving your upper body down and forward. Exhale when moving

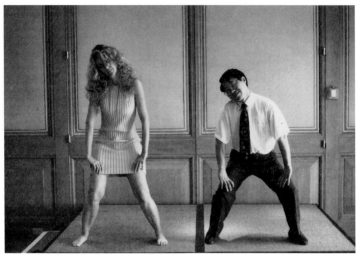

*Figure 7.14: Neck rolls forward. TREASURE 5.*

the body back and around to the front – starting position (Fig. 7.17).

Do four clockwise and four counter-clockwise rotations, making a set of eight. Remember to keep your mind focused on the Qi in the lower Dan Tian.

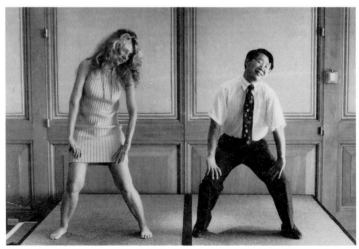

*Figure 7.15: Neck rolls back. TREASURE 5.*

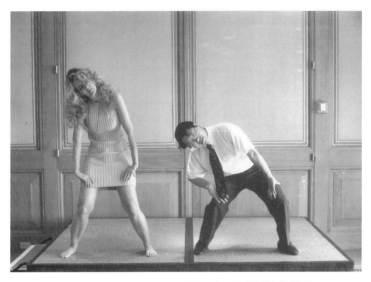

*Figure 7.16: Body rolls side to back. TREASURE 5.*

*Figure 7.17: Body rolls around. TREASURE 5.*

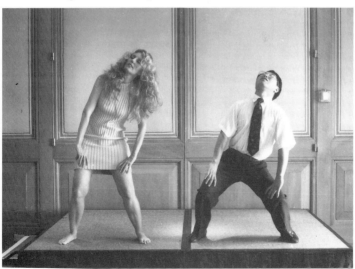

# TREASURE #6:
## Connecting the Heart and Kidneys

*Focus:* In the Sixth Treasure you are strengthening internal energy, balancing the yin and yang, by directing Qi through the heart and kidney meridians. You move your energy in a big cycle, through the triple warmer, through your outstretched arms to the center of your hands (heart meridian). Bending forward you move and connect the Qi to the soles and inner sides of your feet (kidney meridian), up your legs to the lower Dan Tian. The bending forward motion also massages and strengthens the kidneys.

*Posture:* Stand with feet parallel or placed to comfort level, shoulder-width apart, and let your whole body relax. Your arms rest gently at your sides. (See Fig. 7.9 shown previously.)

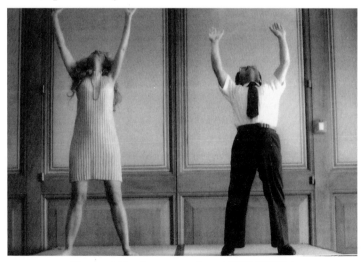

*Figure 7.18: Arm extension. TREASURE 6*

*Movement:* Take a deep breath and relax. Inhale while moving the Qi upward, through the triple warmer, and gently raise the arms forward and upward, over your head. Keep elbows relaxed as you extend the arms over your head, palms facing the sky. Continue to bring the Qi up through the shoulders and arms to the center of the hands. (Fig. 7.18)

Next, bend forward and slowly lower the arms toward the feet, bringing energy down through both hands to reach the inner sides and soles (center) of your feet (Fig. 7.19). Hold this position about five seconds. Slowly straighten your back and return to the starting position. Inhale when raising your arms, exhale while lowering your arms, and gently hold your breath when returning to the starting position.

Complete this movement eight times.

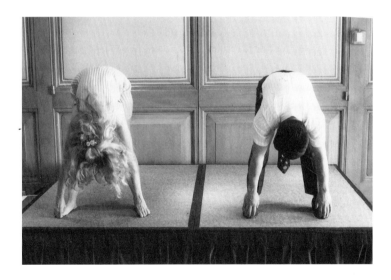

*Figure 7.19: Bring energy to the feet. TREASURE 6*

# TREASURE #7:
## Strengthening Inner Power

*Focus:* In the Seventh Treasure you are developing and using internal and external energy, balancing the flow of yin and yang. This Treasure is more powerful, involving stronger movements, for you are strengthening your inner power. You guide the flow of Qi from the lower Dan Tian up through your arms and hands, accumulating Qi and developing strength.

This Treasure has two segments, the yang and the yin. In the yang segment, you send Qi through the arms and hands by a forceful thrust, or punch. You use your whole body's energy when you thrust or extend your arms.

In the yin segment you send out Qi as you gently extend the arms.

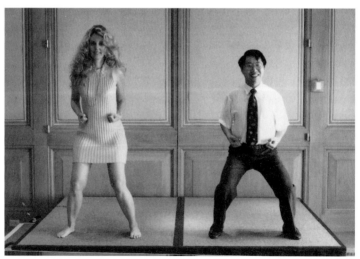

*Figure 7.20: Beginning posture for TREASURE 7*

### *YANG SEGMENT*

*Posture:* Stand in horse stance position, feet about two and one half foot lengths apart, wider than the shoulders. Bend knees. Make fists with each hand, palms up, and place your fists at waist. (Fig. 7.20)

*Movement:* Take a deep breath, guiding the energy up through the triple warmer into your arms and hands, letting the energy accumulate in your hands. With the right fist turning down, punch the right arm forward, expelling the breath (Fig. 7.21), and then return fist to your waist. Repeat to left, punching the left fist and arm forward, expelling the breath (Fig. 7.22), returning the fist to waist.

Repeat to each side. Punch right arm to the right side (Fig. 7.23) and return. Punch left arm to the left side (Fig. 7.24) and return. At each thrust outward, expel the breath with the the sound "huh" from the Qi in the lower Dan Tian, not from the throat. Inhale to begin, exhale and open your eyes when thrusting forward on each punch. Hold the breath to return. Complete two sets of forward and side punches, four punches to a set.

### *YIN SEGMENT*

*Posture:* Stand with legs wide apart in the horse stance position, elbows bent and hands at the lower Dan Tian (Refer back to Fig. 7.3, page 109.)

*Movement:* Take a deep breath, guiding energy up

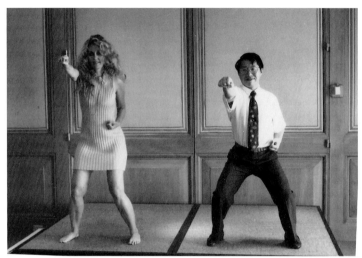

*Figure 7.21: Forward right arm punch. TREASURE 7.*

from the Dan Tian through the triple warmer into arms and hands, letting the energy accumulate in your hands. Raise your arms, extending them to the front, palms facing. Inhale, bringing energy up (Fig. 7.25). Exhale, send energy out and return the arms to their starting position.

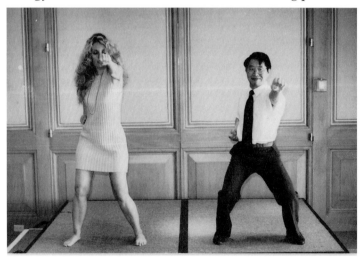

*Figure 7.22  Forward left arm punch.  TREASURE 7.*

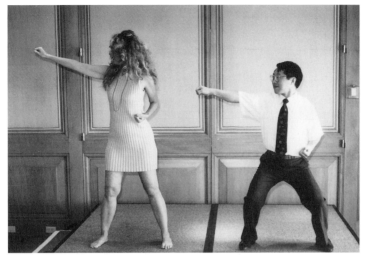

*Figure 7.23: Side right arm punch. TREASURE 7.*

Next, while inhaling, extend both arms to the sides, palms out. Turn your head to the right, exhaling and moving energy through your arms and hands. Turn head to the front, and return arms to the sides.

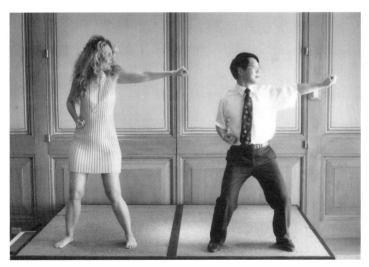

*Figure 7.24 Side left arm punch. TREASURE 7.*

127

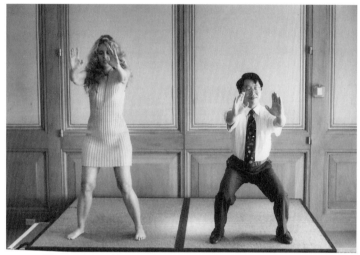

*Figure 7.25: Forward arm extension. TREASURE 7.*

Repeat the front and side movements, turning the head to the left. (Fig. 7.26) A complete set is four movements. Inhale as you begin, and exhale as you extend the arms and return. Complete two sets for a total of eight movements.

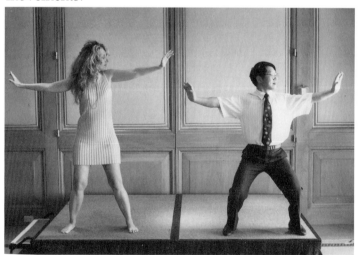

*Figure 7.26: Side arm extension, head left. TREASURE 7.*

# TREASURE #8:
## Settling the Life Force Energy

*Focus:* In the Eighth Treasure you are settling and balancing internal Qi. Pull the energy up to the top of the head, then let it settle back down to the lower Dan Tian. This settles the life force energy through the whole body, allowing the Qi to balance itself and improve all functions.

*Posture:* Stand relaxed with feet parallel or placed to comfort level, shoulder-width apart. Place your arms in back of your body. Women lightly grasp the wrist of the left arm with the right hand, thumb on the inside of the wrist. (Fig. 7.27) Men lightly grasp the wrist of the right

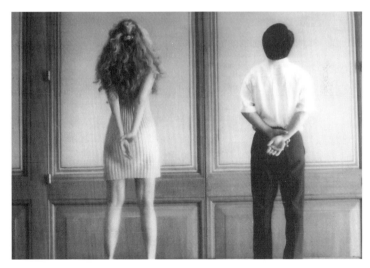

*Figure 7.27: Beginning hand position. TREASURE 8*

arm with the left hand, thumb on inside of the wrist.

*Movement:* Take a deep breath and relax. Focus your mind in the lower Dan Tian. While inhaling, begin guiding the Qi with your mind up through the triple warmer to the top of your head. At the same time, slightly raise heels off the ground, gently balancing on the balls of your feet and begin to loosen grasp on wrist. (Fig. 7.28). Quickly and simultaneously drop your heels to the ground, swing your arms to the front and expel the breath, making a "huh" sound (Fig. 7.29). This sound should come from deep within the lower Dan Tian, not the throat. Allow the Qi to settle back through your body to the lower Dan Tian. Inhale as you move the energy up to the top of the head, exhale as you release your focus on the energy and swing the arms to the front. Let the body adjust the energy by itself. Complete movement seven times.

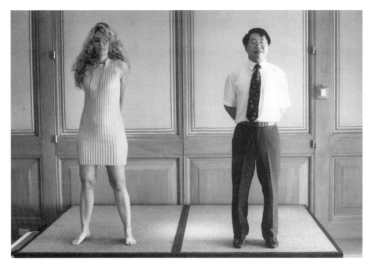

*Figure 7.28: Guiding energy to top of the head. TREASURE 8*

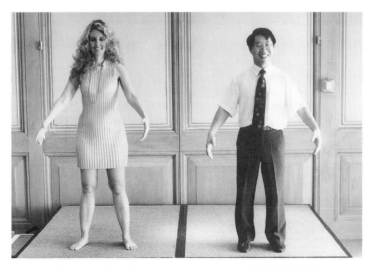

*Figure 7.29: Releasing the energy. TREASURE 8*

# Summary

When you focus on the harmonious order of your own being, all else takes care of itself. Through practicing The Eight Treasures Program, the yin and yang forces maintain balance within your own system; and you begin to realize beneficial effects almost immediately. Your organs will benefit from the very first time you practice these movements. Pain and fatigue will begin to decrease or disappear. You will notice your mental clarity improving because you have more energy. In addition, you may observe other phenomena, such as, heat, lightness, greater intuitive awareness, experiencing your energy field in a new way, seeing lights or an iridescent glow. These are all natural as you learn to develop and experience your Qi.

Don't look for signs. Don't look for anything. Whatever experiences do or don't come to you will be in perfect keeping with what you need as you balance your energy and gain greater strength and vitality. The more you practice and develop a tranquil mind, the more the energy effortlessly moves throughout your body. Remember everyone is different. You will experience feeling better, calmer and happier. Enjoying your life more and more everyday through healthful, confident living is what is really important.

The Eight Treasures of Qigong Program ©

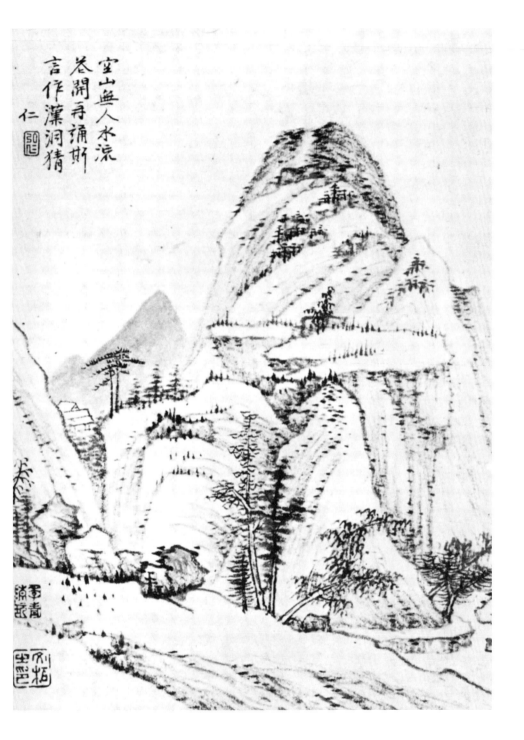

空山無人水流
蒼開尋誦斯
言作藻洞猜
仁

*Conical Peaks and Table-rocks*
Hung Jen (1610-1664)

# CHAPTER 8

# QIGONG MEDITATIONS

*The great Tao produces, maintains
and reproduces all changes in the universe.*

## Developing and Balancing Qi

These Qigong meditations are designed to help focus
the mind, expand awareness of Qi, and develop the life
force within. They promote physical, mental and spiritual
well-being.

These are active meditations. You are working with
the Qi through sensing and visualization, guiding it with
the mind to different meridians and areas of the body.
At the close of the first two meditation exercises, you also
use massage and tapping techniques to stimulate Qi.

These are advanced meditations and have highly
beneficial effects, yet they are easy to do and quite

enjoyable. Although specific postures are suggested, the meditations may be done sitting, standing or reclining, depending upon your circumstances and needs.

As with The Eight Treasures Program, there are no hard rules – no absolutely correct way to do a posture or visualize or experience the energy.

When practicing, give yourself the freedom to follow natural body movements. Don't try to control every little movement. You may experience a variety of sensations, such as, heat, warmth, electricity, cold, fullness, a light breeze – the possibilities are numerous. It is the Qi you are feeling and each individual's responses and sensations are different. It is just like when you collect energy from the earth, the ocean, the sky, the sun, and the universe – that's the Qi energy. This energy can be experienced through each of the physical senses or transcend physical awareness.

Remember – it all comes by itself.

You don't have to look for sensations or special experiences. In fact, anticipation gets in the way of being focused and relaxed during practice. The more you practice, the more the mind and body are sensitized to Qi and the more you understand.

These meditations help you to help yourself physically, mentally and spiritually. The important thing in life is to do whatever you can to help build and balance Qi, for then you can help yourself and others. After practicing these meditations for a while, the inner Qi will guide you. Allow yourself to flow with it.

# Sitting Meditation
## To Strengthen The Internal Organs

In this meditation you use the Qi in the lower Dan Tian to strengthen the internal organs, especially the kidney area, while balancing the yin and yang. You also develop the third eye or psychic energy.

1. Sit comfortably on the floor, legs crossed and back straight. You also may sit in a chair, back straight, if that is more comfortable. Bend your arms at the elbows and put your hands together in a prayer position, palms together and fingers pointing upward, at the level of your heart or chest . (Fig. 8.0)

2. Close your eyes. Touch the tip of the tongue to the roof of your mouth. (It's just a touch and should feel natural and comfortable.) Take three slow, smooth, deep breaths, inhaling through the nose and exhaling through the mouth. Breathe from the lower Dan Tian area.
Relax.

3. Inhale, bringing the energy up from the Dan Tian to the third eye. Use the third eye like a flashlight. Shine it down to the tip of your nose. Now shine the light, the Qi, to the tip of the tongue, through the neck, chest, heart, lungs, stomach, liver, spleen, down to your kidneys, back to the Dan Tian. (You simply move the light energy down through the upper body to the Qi reservoir below the navel.)

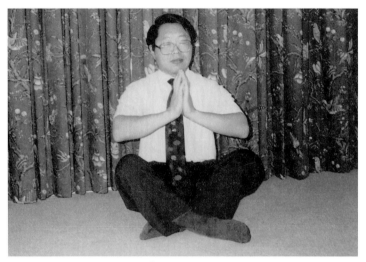

*Figure 8.0: Sitting meditation position*

4. Now picture a calm, clear lake or pool of water in your lower stomach; radiant fire in the upper stomach; and a beautiful flower in your heart.

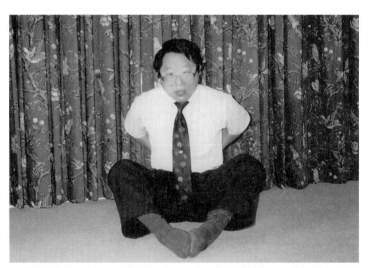

*Figure 8.1: Massaging the lower back and kidneys, front view*

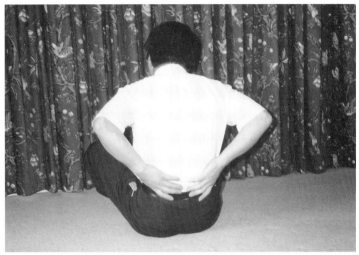

*Figure 8.2: Massaging the lower back and kidneys, back view*

5. The fire in your stomach now moves up through the chest, to the shoulders, the upper body, and flows through the arms to your hands. Hold the fire in your hands and feel the hands getting very hot. Imagine the center of your palms burning like a fireplace.

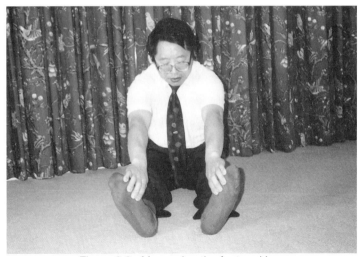

*Figure 8.3: Massaging the feet and legs*

6. Let the energy flow back through the arms and shoulders, up through the neck and head. Let the energy go out the top of your head. Imagine it flowing out. Just release it.

7. Open your arms, inhaling, then close, bringing the arms together, exhaling, keeping the arms approximately at chest level. Breathe in and out, moving the arms in and out, eight times. You are building energy and letting heat build in your hands. The hands may feel very hot. This is the accumulation of Qi.

8. Stretch your legs out in front of you. Let the Qi from your hands flow into the body and energy meridians as you begin to massage yourself. Rub your kidneys, your lower back, up and down, or around in a circle (Figs. 8.1 and 8.2). Then rub the energy on the outside of the legs down to the inside and soles of the feet (Fig. 8.3). You are following the meridian on the outside of your legs down to the inside of your feet. Rub the energy on the sides of your feet and the soles of your feet. Now moving up from the feet, massage the inside of your legs, moving back up to the kidneys in the lower back.

9. Repeat this process three times, rubbing from the lower back, down the outside of your legs, to the inside of your feet, up the inside of your legs to the lower back. Then take a deep breath and relax your body, enjoying the Qi energy.

# Standing Meditation
## To Stimulate The Microcosmic Orbit

This meditation focuses on the spine and the two major energy channels in the upper body. The *Du Mai*, or Governing Vessel, originates at the pelvic floor and travels up the spine to the top of the head, through the third eye and tip of the nose to the inside of the mouth. There it meets the *Ren Mai*, or Conception Vessel, which runs from inside the mouth along the front of the body to the perineum. Touching the tip of the tongue to the roof of the mouth connects the energy and flow between the two vessels. (See Figs. 3.2, 3.3, 3.6, and 3.7.)

This meditation stimulates these major Qi meridians or vessels. All the energies meet at the top of your head, the *Bai Hui*, and nourish the brain. The Governing and Conception Vessels are the most important to be stimulated in maintaining your good health, for they are the main rivers through which the Qi flows out into all the other tributaries, nourishing the organs, systems, cells and tissues.

In this meditation you concentrate on circling the energy, moving it up, down and around through your body, balancing the yin and yang. Every individual is unique and the points may be slightly different, so just move the energy around in a big circle. Don't be concerned about whether you are doing it "exactly right." Do natural breathing, relax, and allow the energy to move through your body.

1. Stand relaxed, feet comfortably apart, and slightly bend the knees. You may either hold the arms down and slightly away from the body; or hold them out to your sides, palms facing up, elbows slightly bent (Fig. 8.4). Eyes may be opened or closed.

2. Touch the tip of your tongue to the roof of the mouth. (It's just a touch, and should feel natural and comfortable.) Take three slow, smooth, deep breaths, inhaling through the nose and exhaling through the mouth. Breathe from the lower Dan Tian. Relax.

3. Imagine that your feet are growing into the earth like roots, and that a beam of light, like a great rope, is extending from the top of your head into the sky. The roots are deeply and solidly holding you on the ground, and the rope of light is holding up your head.

4. Inhale deeply. As you inhale, tighten your rectum, (anal/sphincter lock) pulling the energy up through the rectum, up through the spine, kidney area, upper back, base of the neck, to the top of the head. After tightening the rectum when beginning the exercise, concentrate on moving the energy through the spine, then release the lock.

5. Exhaling, move the energy down to your third eye, to the tip of the nose, tip of the tongue, down through the neck to your heart and chest, back to the Dan Tian. Inhale deeply and strengthen the Qi in the Dan Tian.

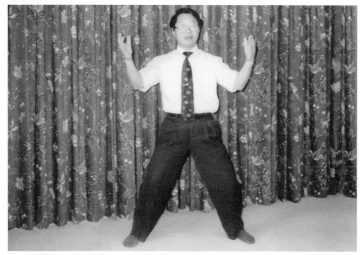

*Figure 8.4: Standing meditation position*

Repeat Steps #4 and #5 two more times, inhaling as you move the energy to the top of the head, and exhaling when returning it to the Dan Tian.

6. With eyes opened, begin inhaling while moving your arms out to the sides at shoulder level, palms facing in; then exhale while moving them back in front of your body at shoulder level, palms facing each other. Repeat this eight times, feeling the heat build in your hands.

7. Begin stimulating the Qi by tapping the inside of your left palm with your right fingers, tapping as you move up the inside of the left arm to the chest. Tap the chest area, the heart area, the shoulder, back down the outside of your arm. Repeat on the other side, tapping with your left fingers. Complete four times.

8. Rub your hands together, feeling the Qi in your hands. Lightly rub the Qi energy on your face and head, back and front of your neck. Take a deep breath and relax, enjoying the Qi energy.

## Rejuvenation Meditation

In this meditation imagine going back to the time when you were a child, when your original Qi energy was very strong and flowing freely. You then bring this vibrant energy back across the years to your present chronological age. You are building internal energy, balancing the yin and yang, awakening memories of vitality, and drawing upon expanded energy resources.

1. Stand in a comfortable position, knees slightly bent, back straight. Extend and round your arms in front of your body, as if you are holding a giant ball of energy (Fig. 8.5). Touch the tip of your tongue to the roof of your mouth and take three deep breaths, inhaling through your nose and exhaling through your mouth, relaxing the tongue. Breathe from the lower Dan Tian. Let your whole body relax. Your eyes may be opened or closed.

2. Imagine you are going back to a time when you were a child. Men go back to age six, and women go back to age seven. Imagine you are a happy child, or remember or create a happy moment. This is a time when your natural Qi is strong and vital. Imagine you are this young child while continuing this meditation.

3. Inhale, and move the Qi from the lower Dan Tian, the great reservoir of energy, up through the triple warmer, through the neck to the top of your head, and down to your third eye.

4. Exhale as you flash your third eye like a flashlight, down to the tip of your nose, the tip of your tongue, down through the neck, chest, heart, lungs, stomach, liver, spleen, kidneys, to the lower Dan Tian. Deposit the energy into your Dan Tian.

Repeat steps #3 and #4 seven times, inhaling as you move the energy up, exhaling on the return.

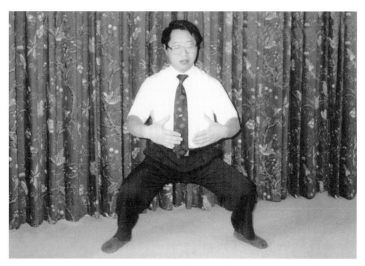

*Figure 8.5: Rejuvenation meditation; holding a giant ball of energy*

5. Open your eyes, and begin slowly opening and closing the arms at chest level. Inhale opening the arms, exhale closing them. Let the energy build in your hands. You may experience your hands feeling warmer and warmer. You might imagine a big ball of energy between your hands. Repeat arm movement eight times.

6. Imagine you have restored your natural health and awareness of this fresh, revitalizing Qi energy. You may complete this meditation in one or two ways: (1) As you slowly open and close your arms several more times, imagine you are swiftly and gently moving through the years to your present age; or (2) Move your arms in and out for every year of your life up to your chronological age, imagining the energy growing stronger with each passing year.

When you reach your present age you feel revitalized, full of youthful energy, enthusiasm, health and vitality. Take a deep breath and relax, letting the Qi settle in the lower Dan Tian. Enjoy the feeling of renewed energy and strength throughout your body, mind and spirit.

## Healing Meditation

A variation of the previous meditations is a special healing meditation for others. If you have been doing the Sitting Meditation, complete Steps 1-7; for the Standing Meditation, complete Steps 1-6; and if following the Rejuvenation Meditation, complete Steps 1-5. You have stimulated the internal Qi in the body and built up the healing energy in your hands. Now you are ready to practice sending the healing energy.

Whether you mentally or physically send healing to someone, he or she will receive it. The more you develop and nurture your own Qi, the stronger your power to emit healing energy to others becomes.

1. Picture the person (or persons) to receive healing energy. See the person as clearly as possible standing or sitting in front of you. If visualization is difficult, just think about caring for the person. (If the person is actually present, of course, place him or her in front of you and proceed.)

2. Extend your arms out and around your image of this person. Send Qi energy through your hands. Move the arms in and out slightly while radiating energy to the person you have pictured. You might imagine the energy flowing as fire or a stream of light to the person, or just sense the energy in your hands.

3. Imagine the person as cheerful, healthy and strong, then release the image or thoughts.

4. Let the Qi build once again in your hands. Direct energy to your own body, mind and spirit. Massage, tap, or rub your own body with healing energy.

# Summary

These meditations help you learn to develop, balance and strengthen Qi. They help you to heighten awareness and learn to deeply relax spiritually, mentally and physically. Then the Qi can flow freely throughout your being, to every cell and tissue and system. You will enjoy the serenity, happiness and love inside your body, and be happier, healthier and more confident in your everyday life. (See Figs. 8.6, 8.7 and 8.8 for additional meditation postures.)

In Chinese philosophy the Tao is the law of heaven and earth. It is the great cosmic principle from which all emerges. Two primary polar forces, the yin and the yang, flow from the Tao. Through their interplay all creation comes into being, is sustained, and passes away. When the yin and the yang are in harmony, all things follow a definite order and unfold smoothly.

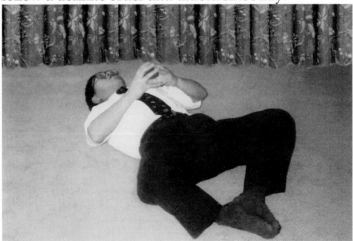

*Figure 8.6: Alternate reclining meditation position, soles together, fingertips together*

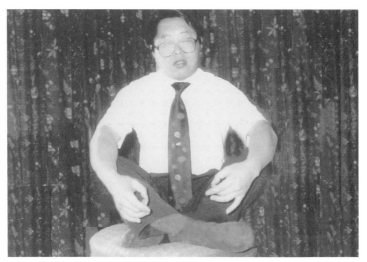

*Figure 8.7: Alternate sitting meditation position; back straight, legs crossed, hands relaxed. Thumb and middle finger form a circle on each hand.*

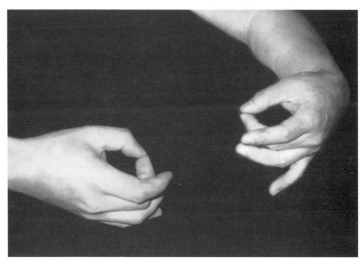

*Figure 8.8: Alternate sitting meditation position. Close-up of hand position*

151

The yin and yang within your own system must be balanced, or else illness can result. This dynamic fluid state of our bodies is what allows us to build and renew our health everyday, and Qigong teaches us how to do just that. Qigong helps us take direct responsibility for our health through using the mind, deep breathing and gentle movements. All we need remember is to practice.

One of the great benefits of Qigong is not only do you build your own health, but you increase your capacity to help others. The stronger your Qi energy is, the more you are able to focus the mind and direct its power. Your ability will then be greater to send healing energy to loved ones, friends or to anyone in need. We find our great joy in life when we develop our own abilities and truly help the world.

*Return to the cradle of creativity, the Tao.*

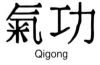

Qigong

# APPENDIX I:
## Glossary Of Selected Terms

*Those who say don't know,*
*and those who know don't say.*

*– Lao-Tzu*

**Acupuncture:** Traditional Chinese healing art in which key points (acupuncture points) along the body's energy meridians are stimulated with fine needles. This therapeutic technique helps restore the balance of yin/yang energy within the body. Acupuncture is used to correct specific disorders, in addition to maintaining overall well-being.

**Dan Tian:** *The Elixir of Life or Elixir Field.* The three locations, areas or fields in your body which house and generate the Qi energy or life force (Elixir). The lower Dan Tian is located internally about three inches below the navel; the middle Dan Tian is located around the stomach, spleen and liver area; and the upper Dan Tian is located in the chest, neck and head region.

**Focus:** Concentration of mental energy. Concentration is an important key to performing Qigong. Concentration or focus usually begins at the lower Dan Tian below the navel, from which one will draw energy to distribute throughout the body. As the energy expands and spreads, so too will the focus. The stronger the focus, the more control one has over the energy and its placement in the body.

**Horse Stance:** A standing posture used often in Qigong. Place feet about two and one half foot lengths apart, wider than your shoulders, and bend the knees, achieving a solid, balanced footing. (See page 109.)

**Meridians:** Passageways or channels within the body through which Qi energy flows. It is estimated there are over 71 meridians forming a great interconnective pattern of energy throughout the body. The energy flowing through the meridians supplies power to the entire system, maintaining balance and energy exchanges with the organs and all bodily functions. Meridians may be thought of as power lines through which mind and spirit can guide and assist the Qi flow in the body.

**Posture:** Position or stance assumed to perform movements in Qigong. Every person is different and has his or her own physical requirements and comfort zones. Therefore, there are no correct or incorrect postures. The postures shown in this book are from classic Qigong. They are age-old basic positions which can be modified (sitting, standing or lying down) to meet individual need and achieve the greatest results.

**Qi:** *(Pronounced Chee)* The vital life force that connects and sustains body, mind and spirit. This life energy is part of and flows from the Tao, the unitive principle of all life. Qi is mainly stored internally in the lower Dan Tian area, approximately three inches below the navel.

**Qigong:** Traditional Chinese self-healing art that helps balance, energize, and strengthen. Qigong, an ancient healing discipline which helps you to sense the energy, restore and maintain health. It is sometimes called *acupuncture without needles* and is an important component of Chinese medicine. Mental focusing, rhythmic breathing and elegant, simple movements characterize this gentle art.

**Tai Chi:** A Chinese system emerging from Qigong that emphasizes flowing movements, meditation and the development of self-discipline. Tai Chi is designed to increase physical flexibility and overall well-being.

**Tao:** The ancient Chinese principle of all life, the unitive law of heaven and earth. The teachings about the Tao are attributed to Lao-Tzu, a Chinese sage. Loosely translated Tao means the way. It is the way of ultimate reality, the unseen life force, father and mother of all creation.

**Taoism:** Ancient Chinese religious and philosophic tradition based on Lao-Tzu's teachings of how to live one's life in harmony with the Tao, or way of the universe. It's underlying belief is that *everything is energy.* The roots of Qigong are found in Taoism, which emphasizes achieving longevity and living a life of balance, health and happiness in harmony with the Tao.

**Third Eye:** Energy center located internally above the bridge of the nose, between the eyebrows in the center of the forehead. Developing the third eye heightens overall perception, awakening one's psychic and intuitive abilities. Through this center, one can learn to receive the finer vibrations of the physical world and attune to realms of subtle energies or forces. Although not recognized by Western science, the third eye is real and vital to our total well-being, especially awakening spiritual consciousness.

**Triple Warmer:** The three energy areas of the inner main torso and head. These areas store and generate Qi: the lower Dan Tian (navel area), middle Dan Tian (solar plexus), and upper Dan Tian (upper body).

**Yin /Yang:** Two polar forces flowing from the Tao which maintain the balance of life, nature and the universe. The yin/yang balance manifests itself through such conditions as female/male, cold/hot, dark/bright, passive/active, stillness/motion. Yet, within each yin force or element is some yang and within every yang force is some yin. They appear separate yet are part of one another, creating the dynamic interplay of life. This universal balancing of opposites maintains harmony and order.

**Yoga:** An ancient method of training in the Hindu tradition designed to unite or integrate body, mind and spirit. The word *Yoga* comes from Sanskrit and means to *yoke* or join. The various forms of Yoga offer different ways to achieve God realization or enlightenment, joining the human spirit with the Divine. Hatha Yoga, which involves physical postures, is the best known and most widely practiced in the West. The other basic Yogas include Jnana Yoga (knowledge), Bhakti Yoga (love or devotion), and Karma Yoga (work or service). Each have their own meditational and philosophical orientations.

# APPENDIX II:
## Questions and Answers About
## The Eight Treasures of Qigong Program©

*1.  What can I expect from learning The Eight Treasures?*

The Eight Treasures Program is designed to embrace all aspects of your life: physically, mentally, spiritually and emotionally. It is a self-healing breathing art which enables each individual to realize and utilize his or her own gift of energy to the fullest potential for total well being.

*2.  Is it easy to learn?*

This program is extremely simple to learn. These graceful movements, which are patterned after nature, are non-structured and flexible. They may be adapted to suit individuality, physical requirements and comfort levels. Mind, breathing and movements are gently combined to help you unite and exchange universal energy within, through and around your being. It is not necessary to know why it works; just that it works.

*3.  How long does it take to learn?*

It takes approximately three to four hours to learn the whole series of movements, depending upon the individual.

*4.  Who can or cannot do it?*

Anyone can do Qigong. It is usually taught in a standing position, but it is equally effective in sitting or even lying down positions. As long as one can breathe and gently focus one's mind, Qigong can be practiced. It is a highly beneficial "energy program" for people of ALL ages, with or without health problems.

5. *How long does it take and how often do you need to practice?*

Although 15 minutes a day is all it takes, practice time can be adjusted to your own schedule. This is a highly flexible program whereby practicing even one treasure for several minutes can be of tremendous benefit. In addition, some people may prefer performing the movements at a slower pace which would extend practice time. Daily practice, however, is the key to success.

6. *Is it necessary to practice with a teacher?*

Once you have learned the program, you can practice independently. Some people prefer to practice in a group as well. Although Qigong supports individual practice, there is an additional benefit to practicing in the presence of a master. A Qigong master is able to raise your level of energy and help guide you towards your own self-empowerment.

7. *What do you need to wear, and where do you practice?*

Qigong requires only that you are comfortable. Just about any type of clothing may be worn during practice. Although Qigong can be performed almost anywhere, many people prefer to practice outside when weather and circumstances permit. It works everywhere.

8. *Generally, what is the difference between Qigong and other energy disciplines?*

Qigong is extremely simple to learn and very easy to do. There is basically no right or wrong way to do it. It is just done with some general guidelines, always emphasizing respect for individual needs. This is a totally non-impact exercise system and can be performed by people with great or minimal agility. Maximum health benefits are always at your fingertips with Qigong.

The purpose of this program is to access and receive energy in a balanced way. How you use it is your decision. Not only will it influence every area of your life in a completely positive and often dramatic way, but it will also open up new horizons to a full spectrum of total well-being.

*Some things are easier said than done.*
*Qigong is easier done than said.*

*Qigong International® was founded in 1993 for the purpose of caring with compassion for each and every individual. It is dedicated to the treatment and prevention of disease and to the promotion of world health care. By helping to create public awareness of the body's natural ability to heal itself through The Eight Treasures of Qigong Program and Qigong Meditations, Dr. Dean Y. Deng and Enid Ballin have established healing practices and educational workshop programs throughout the nation. These programs have proven and continue to be among the easiest and most effective paths to health and total well-being for thousands of people.*

*Acknowledged by hundreds of generations to be the heart of Traditional Chinese Medicine, Qigong reaches back 5,000 years for its genesis. It is considered by some to be the most powerful and sophisticated energy modality in China. This ancient Chinese bio-energy and healing system gains ever increasing acceptance as it integrates with the mainstream consciousness of the western world. This extraordinary echo from the past once again sounds its call for regeneration and reasserts its promise for a brighter, healthier, more fulfilling future for all.*

*Qigong International® is pleased to be a part of this grand reawakening and is excited and happy to share with everyone the unlimited benefits created by the phenomena that is Qigong.*

162

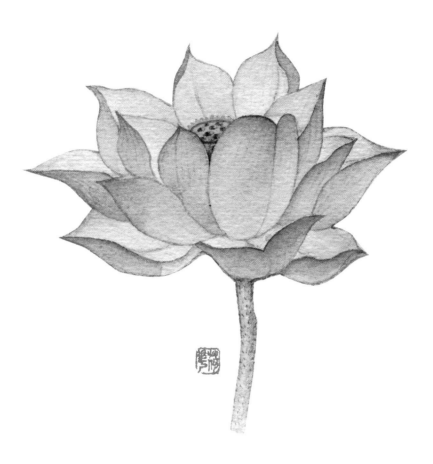

*The Lotus*
Li Zhong Hai

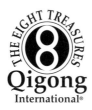

**Qigong**
International®

If you or your organization are interested
in furthering your Qigong experience
through workshops, seminars or
presentations, please contact
QIGONG INTERNATIONAL®
for scheduling information
and arrangements.

Call for information about ordering
*The Eight Treasures of Qigong*
videos, booklets and other
catalog selections.

Also available, direct ordering of
the full length Qigong book
***Qigong, A Legacy In Chinese Healing***
by Dean Y. Deng, M.D.
and Enid Ballin, C.I.E.T.
$18.50
($4.50 ADDITIONAL FOR SHIPPING/HANDLING)

# Qigong International®
## 1-800-821-8324

P.O. Box 56665
New Orleans, LA 70156